Medi

Cookbook

Top Mediterranean Recipes with Low Salt, Low Fat and Less Oil

Danielle Berry

BOOKS UNION
books for life

Table of Contents

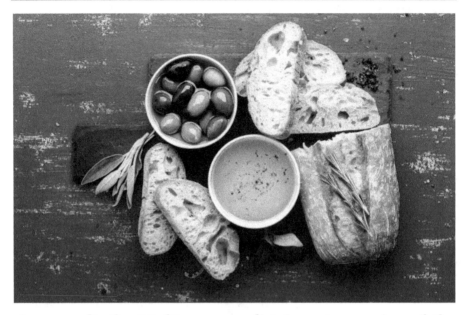

As a result, the Mediterranean diet is an expression of the different food cultures present in the Mediterranean region, with diverse food consumption and production patterns, in continuous evolution representing the particular historical and environmental mosaic that is the Mediterranean. It must be emphasized that there is not one single Mediterranean diet, but rather a several variations on a basic theme adapted to individual country's cultures. Therefore, the Mediterranean diet is more than just a defined diet, but it represents the plurality of various cultural expressions of different Mediterranean food cultures and lifestyles. The term "Mediterranean diet" implies the existence of some common dietary characteristics in Mediterranean countries such as high amounts of olive oil and olives, fruits, vegetables, cereals (mostly unrefined), legumes, and nuts, moderate amounts of fish and dairy products, and low quantities of meat and meat products.

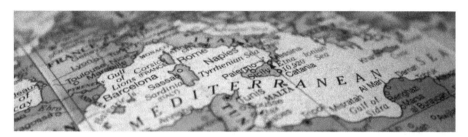

A Mediterranean diet incorporates the traditional healthy living habits of people from countries bordering the Mediterranean Sea, including France, Greece, Italy, and Spain. The Mediterranean diet varies by country and region, so it has a range of definitions. But in general, it's high in vegetables, fruits, legumes, nuts, beans, cereals, grains, fish, and unsaturated fats such as olive oil. It usually includes a low intake of meat and dairy foods. The Mediterranean diet has been linked with good health, including a healthier heart. The way we think about the word "diet" today is as something borne of restriction that helps you lose weight. The Mediterranean diet couldn't be further from that. Rather, it's a heart-healthy eating pattern that includes the food staples of people who live in the countries around the Mediterranean Sea, such as Greece, Croatia, and Italy. right up arrow

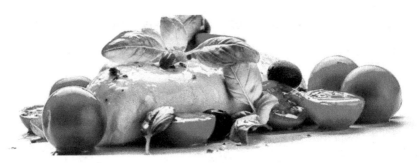

You'll find that in their meals, they emphasize a plant-based eating approach loaded with vegetables and healthy fats, including olive oil and omega-3 fatty acids from fish. It's a diet known for being heart-healthy. right up arrow This diet is rich in fruits and vegetables, whole grains, seafood, nuts and legumes, and olive oil, On this plan, you'll limit or avoid red meat, sugary foods, and dairy (though small amounts like yogurt and cheese are included).

Eating this way means you also have little room for the processed fare. When you look at a plate, it should be bursting with color; traditional proteins like chicken may be more of a side dish compared with produce, which becomes the main event. Mediterranean diet is a generic term based on the traditional eating habits in the countries bordering the Mediterranean Sea. There's not one standard Mediterranean diet. At least 16 countries border the Mediterranean. Eating styles vary among these countries and even among regions within each country because of differences in culture, ethnic background, religion, economy, geography, and agricultural production. However, there are some common factors.

A Mediterranean-Style Diet Typically Includes:

- Plenty of fruits, vegetables, bread and other grains, potatoes, beans, nuts, and seeds;
- Olive oil as a primary fat source; and
- Dairy products, eggs, fish, and poultry in low to moderate amounts.

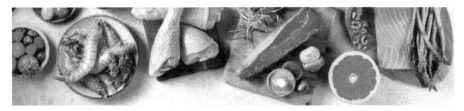

Fish and poultry are more common than red meat in this diet. It also centers on minimally processed, plant-based foods. Wine may be consumed in low to moderate amounts, usually with meals. The fruit is a common dessert instead of sweets.

How To Make Your Diet More Mediterranean

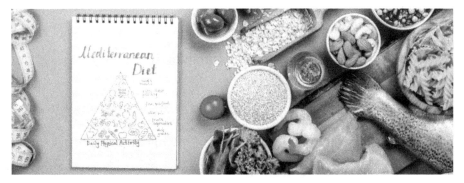

You can make your diet more Mediterranean-style by:

- Eating plenty of starchy foods, such as bread and pasta
- Eating plenty of fruit and vegetables
- Including fish in your diet
- Eating less meat
- Choosing products made from vegetable and plant oils, such as olive oil

The Eatwell Guide

The Mediterranean diet is very similar to the government's healthy eating advice, which is set out in the Eatwell Guide. The guide shows what foods are needed for a healthy, balanced diet and how much you should eat of each food group:

- Eat at least 5 portions of a variety of fruit and vegetables every day – find out more about getting your 5 A Day
- Base your meals on starchy foods such as potatoes, bread, rice, and pasta – choose wholegrain versions where possible
- Eat some beans or pulses, fish, eggs, meat, and other proteins (including 2 portions of fish every week, 1 of which should be oily)
- Have some dairy or dairy alternatives (such as soya drinks) – choose lower-fat and lower-sugar options
- Choose unsaturated oils and spreads, and eat them in small amounts
- Drink 6 to 8 glasses of fluid a day

- If consuming foods and drinks that are high in fat, salt, or sugar, have them less often and in small amounts – find out more about reducing sugar in your diet
- You do not need to achieve this balance with every meal, but try to get it right over a day or even a week.

Does The AHA Recommend A Mediterranean-Style Diet?

Yes. A Mediterranean-style diet can help you achieve the American Heart Association's recommendations for a healthy dietary pattern that:

- Emphasizes vegetables, fruits, whole grains, beans, and legumes;
- Includes low-fat or fat-free dairy products, fish, poultry, non-tropical vegetable oils and nuts; and
- Limits added sugars, sugary beverages, sodium, highly processed foods, refined carbohydrates, saturated fats, and fatty or processed meats.

This style of eating can play a big role in preventing heart disease and stroke and reducing risk factors such as obesity, diabetes, high cholesterol, and high blood pressure. There is some evidence that a Mediterranean diet rich in virgin olive oil may help the body remove excess cholesterol from arteries and keep blood vessels open.

EXPLANATION OF MEDITERRANEAN DIET

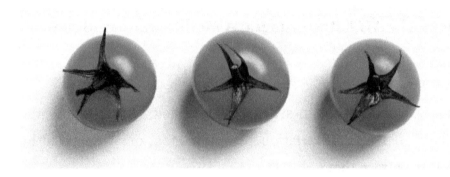

What Is The Mediterranean Diet?

The Mediterranean diet is an eating approach that people who live in regions around the Mediterranean Sea have naturally adopted. It's rich in fresh, whole foods (olive oil, nuts, seeds, veggies, fruit, and fish) and low in red meat and processed fare. It's generally accepted that the folks in countries bordering the Mediterranean Sea live longer and suffer less than most Americans from cancer and cardiovascular ailments. The not-so-surprising secret is an active lifestyle, weight control, and a diet low in red meat, sugar, and saturated fat and high in produce, nuts, and other healthful foods. The Mediterranean Diet may offer a host of health benefits, including weight loss, heart and brain health, cancer prevention, and diabetes prevention and control. By following the Mediterranean Diet, you could also keep that weight off while avoiding chronic disease.

There isn't "a" Mediterranean diet. Greeks eat differently from Italians, who eat differently from the French and Spanish. But they share many of the same principles. Oldways, a nonprofit food think tank in Boston, developed a consumer-friendly Mediterranean diet pyramid that offers guidelines on how to fill your plate and maybe wineglass the Mediterranean way.

What Foods Are Not Allowed On The Mediterranean Diet?

The Mediterranean diet isn't a restrictive fad diet that focuses on eliminating a bunch of foods from your diet. That said, you'll want to limit your intake of foods high in saturated fat, as well as red meat, butter, and dairy milk. You can drink red wine on the Mediterranean diet, but you'll want to do so only in moderation.

What Is A Mediterranean Diet Meal Plan?

Fill half of your plate with fruit and vegetables, and then devote one each of the remaining two quarters to lean proteins and whole grains. Aim to add a serving of low-fat or nonfat dairy, like milk or yogurt, to the side of each meal. Also, enjoying food with friends and family is a tenet of the eating approach.

What Is The Mediterranean Diet?

The Mediterranean diet is a way of eating based on the traditional cuisine of countries bordering the Mediterranean Sea. While there is no single definition of the Mediterranean diet, it is typically high in vegetables, fruits, whole grains, beans, nuts and seeds, and olive oil.

How Does The Mediterranean Diet Work Exactly?

The Mediterranean diet wasn't built like a weight loss plan, because it wasn't developed at all but is a style of eating in a region of people that evolved naturally over centuries, there's no official way to follow it. But it's popular because it's a well-rounded approach to eating that isn't restrictive. Also worth noting is two of the five so-called blue zones areas where people live longer and have lower rates of disease are located in Mediterranean cities (Ikaria in Greece and Sardinia in Italy).

How Does Mediterranean Diet Work?

Because this is an eating pattern – not a structured diet – you're on your own to figure out how many calories you should eat to lose or maintain your weight, what you'll do to stay active, and how you'll shape your Mediterranean menu. The Mediterranean diet pyramid should help get you started. The pyramid emphasizes eating fruits, veggies, whole grains, beans, nuts, legumes, olive oil, and flavorful herbs and spices; fish and seafood at least a couple of times a week; and poultry, eggs, cheese, and yogurt in moderation, while saving sweets and red meat for special occasions. Top it off with a splash of red wine (if you want), remember to stay physically active and you're set. While certainly not required, a glass a day for women and two a day for men is fine if your doctor says so. Red wine has gotten a boost because it contains resveratrol, a compound that seems to add years to life – but you'd have to drink hundreds or thousands of glasses to get enough resveratrol to possibly make a difference.

The Main Components Of The Mediterranean Diet Include:

- Daily consumption of vegetables, fruits, whole grains, and healthy fats
- Weekly intake of fish, poultry, beans, and eggs
- Moderate portions of dairy products
- Limited intake of red meat

Plant-Based, Not Meat-Based

The foundation of the Mediterranean diet is vegetables, fruits, herbs, nuts, beans, and whole grains. Meals are built around these plant-based foods. Moderate amounts of dairy, poultry, and eggs are also central to the Mediterranean Diet, as is seafood. In contrast, red meat is eaten only occasionally.

Healthy fats

Healthy fats are a mainstay of the Mediterranean diet. They're eaten instead of less healthy fats, such as saturated and trans fats, which contribute to heart disease. Olive oil is the primary source of added fat in the Mediterranean diet. Olive oil provides monounsaturated fat, which has been found to lower total cholesterol and low-density lipoprotein (LDL or "bad") cholesterol levels. Nuts and seeds also contain monounsaturated fat. Fish are also important in the Mediterranean diet.

Fatty fish such as mackerel, herring, sardines, albacore tuna, salmon, and lake trout are rich in omega-3 fatty acids, a type of polyunsaturated fat that may reduce inflammation in the body. Omega-3 fatty acids also help decrease triglycerides, reduce blood clotting, and decrease the risk of stroke and heart failure.

What About Wine?

The Mediterranean diet typically allows red wine in moderation. Although alcohol has been associated with a reduced risk of heart disease in some studies, it's by no means risk-free. The Dietary Guidelines for Americans caution against beginning to drink or drinking more often based on potential health benefits.

Eating The Mediterranean Way

Interested in trying the Mediterranean diet? These tips will help you get started:

- **Eat More Fruits And Vegetables:** Aim for 7 to 10 servings a day of fruit and vegetables.
- **Opt For Whole Grains:** Switch to whole-grain bread, cereal and pasta. Experiment with other whole grains, such as bulgur and farro.
- **Use Healthy Fats:** Try olive oil as a replacement for butter when cooking. Instead of putting butter or margarine on bread, try dipping it in flavored olive oil.
- **Eat More Seafood:** Eat fish twice a week. Fresh or water-packed tuna, salmon, trout, mackerel, and herring are healthy choices. Grilled fish tastes good and requires little cleanup. Avoid deep-fried fish.
- **Reduce Red Meat:** Substitute fish, poultry, or beans for meat. If you eat meat, make sure it's lean and keep portions small.
- **Enjoy Some Dairy:** Eat low-fat Greek or plain yogurt and small amounts of a variety of cheeses.
- **Spice It Up:** Herbs and spices boost flavor and lessen the need for salt.

The Mediterranean diet is a delicious and healthy way to eat. Many people who switch to this style of eating say they'll never eat any other way.

What Kind Of Fats Are Allowed On The Mediterranean Diet?

Focus on incorporating monounsaturated fats into your diet. This type of fat can be found in such foods as avocado, nuts, olive oil, and fatty fish, and has been linked to a lower risk of heart disease. Avoid or limit saturated fat, which can cause high cholesterol, and is found in foods such as full-fat dairy and red meat.

The Basics

- Eat Vegetables, fruits, nuts, seeds, legumes, potatoes, whole grains, bread, herbs, spices, fish, seafood, and extra virgin olive oil.
- Eat-in moderation: Poultry, eggs, cheese, and yogurt.
- Eat only rarely: Red meat.
- Don't eat Sugar-sweetened beverages, added sugars, processed meat, refined grains, refined oils, and other highly processed foods.

Avoid These Unhealthy Foods

You should avoid these unhealthy foods and ingredients:

- Added sugar: Soda, candies, ice cream, table sugar, and many others.
- Refined grains: White bread, pasta made with refined wheat, etc.
- Trans fats: Found in margarine and various processed foods.

- Refined oils: Soybean oil, canola oil, cottonseed oil, and others.
- Processed meat: Processed sausages, hot dogs, etc.
- Highly processed foods: Anything labeled "low-fat" or "diet" or which looks like it was made in a factory.

You must read food labels carefully if you want to avoid these unhealthy ingredients.

Foods To Eat

Exactly which foods belong to the Mediterranean diet is controversial, partly because there is such variation between different countries. The diet examined by most studies is high in healthy plant foods and relatively low in animal foods. However, eating fish and seafood is recommended at least twice a week. The Mediterranean lifestyle also involves regular physical activity, sharing meals with other people, and enjoying life. You should base your diet on these healthy, unprocessed Mediterranean foods:

- **Vegetables:** Tomatoes, broccoli, kale, spinach, onions, cauliflower, carrots, Brussels sprouts, cucumbers, etc.
- **Fruits:** Apples, bananas, oranges, pears, strawberries, grapes, dates, figs, melons, peaches, etc.
- **Nuts And Seeds:** Almonds, walnuts, macadamia nuts, hazelnuts, cashews, sunflower seeds, pumpkin seeds, etc.

- **Legumes:** Beans, peas, lentils, pulses, peanuts, chickpeas, etc.
- **Tubers:** Potatoes, sweet potatoes, turnips, yams, etc.
- **Whole Grains:** Whole oats, brown rice, rye, barley, corn, buckwheat, whole wheat, whole-grain bread, and pasta.
- **Fish And Seafood:** Salmon, sardines, trout, tuna, mackerel, shrimp, oysters, clams, crab, mussels, etc.
- **Poultry:** Chicken, duck, turkey, etc.
- **Eggs:** Chicken, quail, and duck eggs.
- **Dairy:** Cheese, yogurt, Greek yogurt, etc.
- **Herbs And Spices:** Garlic, basil, mint, rosemary, sage, nutmeg, cinnamon, pepper, etc.
- **Healthy Fats:** Extra virgin olive oil, olives, avocados, and avocado oil.
- Whole, single-ingredient foods are the key to good health.

What To Drink

- Water should be your go-to beverage on a Mediterranean diet.
- This diet also includes moderate amounts of red wine — around 1 glass per day.
- However, this is completely optional, and wine should be avoided by anyone with alcoholism or problems controlling their consumption.

- Coffee and tea are also completely acceptable, but you should avoid sugar-sweetened beverages and fruit juices, which are very high in sugar.

What Food Can You Eat On Mediterranean Diet?

- Fruits and veggies take up the most space on the Mediterranean food pyramid. Fill up on plant foods at least twice a week, preferably more.
- Olive oil is a cooking staple in Mediterranean recipes and a key salad dressing ingredient.
- Whole grains, beans, nuts, and legumes are always allowed.
- Fish and seafood are recommended at least twice weekly.
- Wine (in moderation and if you drink) and water are typical Mediterranean beverages.

What Foods Should You Limit On Mediterranean Diet?

- Eggs and poultry are occasional foods, in moderate portions.
- Cheese and yogurt are traditional Mediterranean foods, also in moderate portions.

A Mediterranean Sample Menu For 1 Week

Below is a sample menu for one week on the Mediterranean diet. Feel free to adjust the portions and food choices based on your own needs and preferences.

Monday

- Breakfast: Greek yogurt with strawberries and oats.
- Lunch: Whole-grain sandwich with vegetables.
- Dinner: A tuna salad, dressed in olive oil. A piece of fruit for dessert.

Tuesday

- Breakfast: Oatmeal with raisins.
- Lunch: Leftover tuna salad from the night before.
- Dinner: Salad with tomatoes, olives, and feta cheese.

Wednesday

- Breakfast: Omelet with veggies, tomatoes, and onions. A piece of fruit.
- Lunch: Whole-grain sandwich, with cheese and fresh vegetables.
- Dinner: Mediterranean lasagne.

Thursday

- Breakfast: Yogurt with sliced fruits and nuts.
- Lunch: Leftover lasagne from the night before.
- Dinner: Broiled salmon, served with brown rice and vegetables.

Friday

- Breakfast: Eggs and vegetables, fried in olive oil.
- Lunch: Greek yogurt with strawberries, oats, and nuts.
- Dinner: Grilled lamb, with salad and baked potato.

Saturday

- Breakfast: Oatmeal with raisins, nuts, and an apple.
- Lunch: Whole-grain sandwich with vegetables.
- Dinner: Mediterranean pizza made with whole wheat, topped with cheese, vegetables, and olives.

Sunday

- Breakfast: Omelet with veggies and olives.
- Lunch: Leftover pizza from the night before.
- Dinner: Grilled chicken, with vegetables and a potato. Fruit for dessert.

There is usually no need to count calories or track macronutrients (protein, fat, and carbs) on the Mediterranean diet.

Healthy Mediterranean Snacks

You don't need to eat more than 3 meals per day. But if you become hungry between meals, there are plenty of healthy snack options:

- A handful of nuts.
- A piece of fruit.
- Carrots or baby carrots.
- Some berries or grapes.
- Leftovers from the night before.
- Greek yogurt.
- Apple slices with almond butter.

How To Follow The Diet At Restaurants

It's very simple to make most restaurant meals suitable for the Mediterranean diet.

- Choose fish or seafood as your main dish.
- Ask them to fry your food in extra virgin olive oil.
- Only eat whole-grain bread, with olive oil instead of butter.

A Simple Shopping List For The Diet

It is always a good idea to shop at the perimeter of the store. That's usually where the whole foods are. Always try to choose the least processed option. Organic is best, but only if you can easily afford it.

- Vegetables: Carrots, onions, broccoli, spinach, kale, garlic, etc.
- Fruits: Apples, bananas, oranges, grapes, etc.
- Berries: Strawberries, blueberries, etc.
- Frozen veggies: Choose mixes with healthy vegetables.
- Grains: Whole-grain bread, whole-grain pasta, etc.
- Legumes: Lentils, pulses, beans, etc.
- Nuts: Almonds, walnuts, cashews, etc.
- Seeds: Sunflower seeds, pumpkin seeds, etc.
- Condiments: Sea salt, pepper, turmeric, cinnamon, etc.
- Fish: Salmon, sardines, mackerel, trout.
- Shrimp and shellfish.
- Potatoes and sweet potatoes.
- Cheese.
- Greek yogurt.
- Chicken.
- Pastured or omega-3 enriched eggs.
- Olives.
- Extra virgin olive oil.

It's best to clear all unhealthy temptations from your home, including sodas, ice cream, candy, pastries, white bread, crackers, and processed foods. If you only have healthy food in your home, you will eat healthy food.

What Are The Health Benefits Of The Mediterranean Diet?

The Mediterranean diet has been praised for its potential heart benefits. It may also help improve type 2 diabetes management and help with weight loss depending on the foods you choose to eat on this plan.

Why The Mediterranean Diet?

The Mediterranean diet is my favorite way of eating. Let me point out that even though the word diet is thrown in there, it's technically not a diet in the way that we think of weight-loss diets. It's an overall dietary pattern. A very healthy one!

What Are The Potential And Known Health Benefits Of The Mediterranean Diet?

The Mediterranean diet is most famous for its benefit to heart health, decreasing the risk of heart disease by, in part, lowering levels of LDL ("bad") cholesterol and reducing mortality from cardiovascular conditions. It's also been credited with a lower likelihood of certain cancers, like breast cancer, as well as conditions like Parkinson's disease and Alzheimer's disease.

Emerging evidence suggests that eating this way may offer protective effects for those with or at risk for type 2 diabetes. For one, Mediterranean eating improves blood sugar control in those already diagnosed with the condition, suggesting it can be a good way to manage the disease. What's more, given that those with diabetes are at increased odds for cardiovascular disease, adopting this diet can help improve their heart health.

Finally, people eat about nine servings of fruit and vegetables a day on a Mediterranean diet. Produce packs an array of disease-fighting antioxidants, and people who fill their diet with these foods have a lower risk of disease.

What Are The Pros And Cons Of A Mediterranean Diet?

When you're deciding whether a Mediterranean Diet is right for you, consider these pros and cons:

Pros

1. It's Easy To Stick With: A diet works only if it's doable. That means everyone in your family can eat it and you can eat in this style no matter where you go (to a restaurant for dinner, to a family event). With its flavors and variety of foods that don't cut out any food group, this is one such eating plan. It is an appealing diet that one can stay with for a lifetime.

2. You Can Eat What You Love: It's evident that with such a variety of whole, fresh foods available to you as options, it's easy to build meals based on the diet. And you don't have to eliminate your favorites, either. They may require just some tweaks. For instance, rather than a sausage and pepperoni pizza, you'd choose one piled high with veggies. You can also fit a lot of food into one meal. Filling up on fresh foods like fruit and vegetables will allow you to build volume into meals for fewer calories.

3. It's Low In Saturated Fat: You're not going to feel hungry eating this way, because you can build in a variety of healthy fats. But by limiting large amounts of red or processed meats and relying heavily on monounsaturated fatty acids, like avocado, nuts, or olive oil, you'll keep saturated fat levels low. These fats don't lead to high cholesterol the same way saturated fats do. Healthful sources of fat include olive oil, fish oils, and nut-based oils.

4. It Reduces The Risk Of Disease: A growing number of studies suggest that people who follow a Mediterranean diet are less likely to die of heart disease than people who follow a typical American diet. What's more, the evidence is emerging that shows people who eat this way have a lower risk of colon cancer, prostate cancer, and some head and neck cancers.

Cons

1. Milk Is Limited: There are no long-term risks to eating the Mediterranean, But you may be put off if you're big on eating a lot of milk and rely on it to get all the calcium you need. You'll get to eat cheese and yogurt but in smaller amounts. To get enough calcium in the diet without milk, one would need to eat enough yogurt and cheese, or seek non-dairy calcium sources. If needed, drink skim milk. Otherwise, nondairy calcium sources include fortified almond milk, sardines, kale, and tofu made with calcium sulfate. right up arrow

2. You Still Have To Cap Alcohol: The hallmark of a Mediterranean diet is that drinking red wine socially is thought to be one reason why the diet is so healthy. But women should still stick to one glass and men two glasses. If you have a history of breast cancer in the family, know that any alcohol consumption raises that risk. right up arrow, In that case, talk to your doctor to find out what's right for you.

3. Fat Isn't Unlimited Either: As with wine, it's possible to get too much of a good thing when it comes to healthy fats. While the Mediterranean diet meets heart-healthy diet limits for saturated fat, your total fat consumption could be greater than the daily recommended amount if you aren't careful. Plus, as Harvard Health Publishing notes, not all fats are created equal, and you'll want to minimize your saturated fat intake in favor of healthier fats like those found in olive oil. Your total daily fat intake should provide 20 to 35 percent of your total daily caloric intake, according to the Institute of Medicine (now the National Academies of Science, Engineering, and Medicine), and saturated fats should represent less than 7 percent of your total caloric intake.

4. You Have To Find Time To Cook: While you don't have to spend hours in your kitchen, you will need to cook because the diet is all about working with delicious fresh food. You may have a learning curve as you build these skills.

What Are The Potential Short- And Long-Term Effects Of A Mediterranean Diet?

As has become obvious, there are numerous potential benefits from adopting a Mediterranean diet. Over the long term, these health effects may be more pronounced and can include better brain health by slowing cognitive decline and lowering the risk of Alzheimer's disease and other dementias.

It also may help stave off chronic diseases, like heart disease and type 2 diabetes, as well as act protectively against certain cancers. The diet is also a boon to mental health, as it's associated with reduced odds of depression. There's even some data to suggest it can be supportive in relieving symptoms of arthritis.

In the short term, you may lose a modest amount of weight over a year and are likely to keep it off if you continue to eat following the diet. If eating in the Mediterranean style prompts you to consume more fruit and vegetables, you'll not only feel better physically, but your mental health will get a lift, too. Research shows that people who eat more raw fruit and veggies (particularly dark leafy greens like spinach, fresh berries, and cucumber) have fewer symptoms of depression, a better mood, and more life satisfaction.

Will Mediterranean Diet Help You Lose Weight?

The Mediterranean diet might help you lose weight. While some people fear that eating a diet like the Mediterranean diet that is relatively rich in fats (think olive oil, olives, avocado, and some cheese) will keep them fat, more and more research is suggesting the opposite is true. Of course, it depends on which aspects you adopt and how it compares to your current diet. If, for instance, you build a "calorie deficit" into your plan – eating fewer calories than your daily recommended max or burning off extra by exercising – you should shed some pounds. How quickly and whether you keep them off is up to you.

Reasons To Love The Mediterranean Diet

1. Surprise! No Calorie Counting

You won't need a calculator for this meal plan. Instead of adding up numbers, you swap out bad fats for heart-healthy ones. Go for olive oil instead of butter. Try fish or poultry rather than red meat. Enjoy fresh fruit and skip sugary, fancy desserts. Eat your fill of flavorful veggies and beans. Nuts are good but stick to a handful a day. You can have whole-grain bread and wine but in moderate amounts.

2. The Food Is Fresh

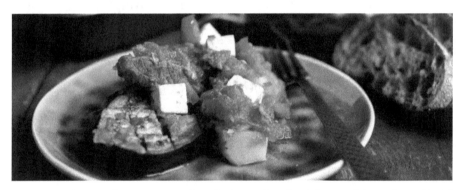

You won't need to roam the frozen food aisle or hit a fast-food drive-thru. The focus is on seasonal food that's made in simple, mouth-watering ways. Build a yummy salad from spinach, cucumbers, and tomatoes. Add classic Greek ingredients like black olives and feta cheese with a Quick Light Greek Salad recipe. You can also whip up a colorful, veggie-filled batch of Grilled Tomato Gazpacho.

3. You Can Have Bread

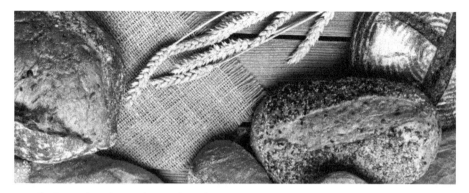

Look for a loaf made with whole grains. It's got more protein and minerals and is generally healthier than the white flour kind. Try whole-grain pita bread dipped in olive oil, hummus, or tahini (a protein-rich paste made from ground sesame seeds).

4. Fat Isn't Forbidden

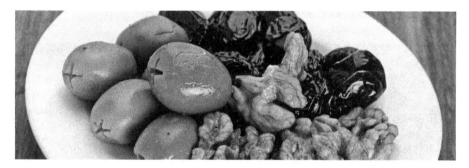

You just need to look for the good kind. You'll find it in nuts, olives, and olive oil. These fats (not the saturated and trans fat hidden in processed foods) add flavor and help fight diseases from diabetes to cancer. Basic Basil Pesto is a tasty way to get some into your diet.

5. The Menu Is Huge

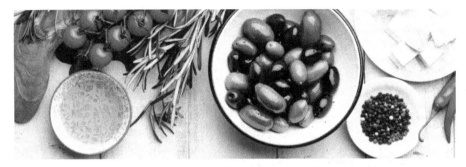

It's more than just Greek and Italian cuisine. Look for recipes from Spain, Turkey, Morocco, and other countries. Choose foods that stick to the basics: light on red meat and whole-fat dairy, with lots of fresh fruits and veggies, olive oil, and whole grains. This Moroccan recipe with chickpeas, okra, and spices fits the healthy Mediterranean profile.

6. The Spices Are Delicious

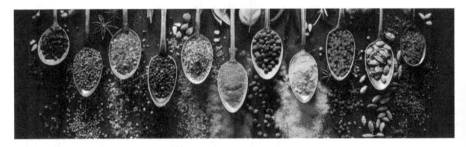

Bay leaves, cilantro, coriander, rosemary, garlic, pepper, and cinnamon add so much flavor you won't need to reach for the salt shaker. Some have health benefits, too. Coriander and rosemary, for example, have disease-fighting antioxidants and nutrients.

This recipe for Greek-Style Mushrooms uses cilantro and coriander and has a lemony kick.

7. It's Easy To Make

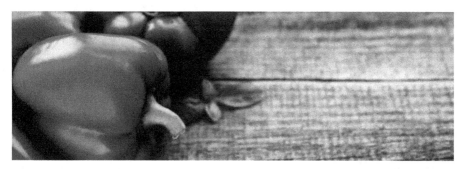

Greek meals are often small, easy to assemble plates called mezze. For your serve-it-cold casual meal, you could put out plates of cheese, olives, and nuts. Also, check out these recipes for Basil Quinoa With Red Bell Pepper and Eight Layered Greek Dip. Both have heart-friendly ingredients including olive oil, beans, whole grains, and spices.

8. You Can Have Wine

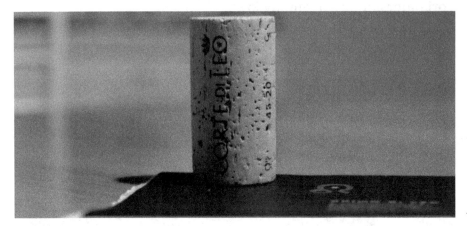

A glass with meals is common in many Mediterranean countries, where dining is often leisurely and social. Some studies suggest that for some people, up to one glass a day for women and two for men may be good for your heart. Red wine may be healthier than white. Check with your doctor to see if it's a good idea for you.

9. You Won't Be Hungry

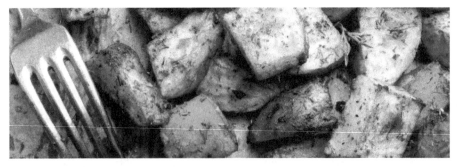

You'll get a chance to eat rich-tasting foods like roasted sweet potatoes, hummus, and even this Lima Bean Spread. You digest them slowly so that you feel full longer. Hunger's not a problem when you can munch on nuts, olives, or bites of low-fat cheese when a craving strikes. Feta and halloumi are lower in fat than cheddar but still rich and tasty.

10. You Can Lose Weight

You'd think it would take a miracle to drop some pounds if you eat nuts, cheese, and oils. But those Mediterranean basics (and the slower eating style) let you feel full and satisfied. And that helps you stick to a diet. Regular exercise is also an important part of the lifestyle.

11. Your Heart Will Thank You

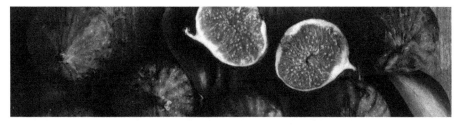

Almost everything in this diet is good for your heart. Olive oil and nuts help lower "bad" cholesterol. Fruits, veggies, and beans help keep arteries clear. Fish helps lower triglycerides and blood pressure. Even a daily glass of wine may be good for your heart! If you've never fallen in love with fish, try this Mediterranean-inspired recipe for Grilled Whole Trout With Lemon-Tarragon Bean Salad.

12. You'll Stay Sharper Longer

The same goodness that protects your heart is also good for your brain. You're not eating bad fats and processed foods, which can cause inflammation. Instead, antioxidant-rich foods make this eating style a brain-friendly choice.

The Mediterranean Diet For Longevity And Healthful Aging Adding Years To Your Life.

The Mediterranean diet is a healthy eating pattern traditional to regions surrounding the Mediterranean Sea, such as Crete, Spain, and Italy. Research looking at this population and longevity does seem to say that the Mediterranean way can keep aging at bay.

In one large study, consumption of a Mediterranean diet resulted in increased telomere length, a biomarker of aging in humans. Although the accuracy of this biomarker is under debate, the results from this study did support others researching the Mediterranean diet and longevity. Multiple large prospective cohort studies, the type that follows participants over many years, have repeatedly shown that higher adherence to the Mediterranean diet is associated with a lower risk of death or all-cause mortality.

What is the quantity of life without quality one might ask? As it turns out, the Mediterranean diet has also been shown to promote healthy aging, which is defined as living to 70 years of age or older with no major chronic diseases and in good physical and mental health. This begs the question: how long do we need to follow a Mediterranean diet to add years to our life? That remains unknown. The good news, however, is that it is never too late to start.

How To Get Started On The Mediterranean Diet.

The benefits associated with the Mediterranean diet cannot be attributed to a single dietary component, but the pattern as a whole. Here is how to get started.

1. Eat An Abundance Of Unprocessed Plant-Based Foods.

This dietary pattern relies heavily on home cooking and plant-based foods. At the base of the Mediterranean, the meal is vegetables, fruit, whole grains, beans, legumes, nuts, herbs, and spices. As a result, this diet is high in fiber as well as in anti-inflammatory and antioxidant plant compounds, known for their protective roles against chronic disease and aging.

2. Consume A High-Fat Diet.

The Mediterranean diet is high in fat, with over 37% of daily calories coming from healthy fats. Cold-pressed, extra-virgin olive oil is the principal source of fat consumed with other sources including nuts, seeds, fatty fish, and seafood.

3. Consume Red Meat And Dairy Only Occasionally.

Traditionally, red meat and dairy are eaten on a weekly or bi-weekly basis. When consumed, these foods are eaten in modest amounts and with a focus on quality local products, such as flavourful artisanal cheeses.

4. Switch To Intact Grains.

Contrary to popular belief, a Mediterranean diet doesn't mean subsisting on pasta and pizza, but rather on whole, intact grains. Bulgur, farro, black rice, barley, and their flours are often used in fresh salads, soups, risottos, or as bases for dishes loaded with vegetables, herbs, and spices.

5. Enjoy meals with friends.

Hospitality, meal sharing, and the family table are foundational components of the Mediterranean diet. Given that social interaction is a known independent contributor to mental health and longevity, this element of the Mediterranean diet, or rather lifestyle, should not be overlooked. Because sharing meals with loved ones may add years to our life, but more importantly, life to our years.

6. It's All About The Lifestyle.

One of the best things about the Mediterranean diet is that it's all about the lifestyle. This eating philosophy originated based on the longevity of people in the Mediterranean, and researchers observed more than just eating habits. Simply eating Mediterranean diet recipes is not all there is to it. Here's what's important in addition to food:

- Stay active and exercise regularly.
- Avoid smoking.
- Reduce the amount of stress in your lifestyle.
- Actively participate in the community: be invested and engaged in the people around you!

These are the same principles that contribute to longevity in the Mediterranean diet.

Top Mediterranean Diet Recipes!

Without further ado, here are our Mediterranean diet recipes! These recipes feature:

- Olive oil is the cooking oil of choice.
- Beans, lentils, bulgur wheat, quinoa, and rice as major players. They've gotten a bad rap with the interest in the keto diet and Whole 30, but recipes in the Mediterranean diet include beans and whole grains as nutritious foods.

- Vegetarian, vegan, gluten-free, salads, dairy-free,vegetables, chickens & seafood recipes. Mediterranean diet recipes are plant-based, but it's recommended to include seafood about 2 times per week.

Mediterranean Diet Recipes

The Mediterranean diet is based on timeworn peasant-style fare eaten by the healthy populations of Greece, Spain, and Southern Italy. Today, following the diet means consuming an abundance of fresh, seasonal vegetables, rounded out with plenty of legumes and minimally processed whole grains, weekly servings of seafood, small amounts of red meat, modest servings of natural milk products, and a healthy intake of extra virgin olive oil. Small quantities of high-antioxidant red wine, nuts, and natural sugar (in the form of honey and daily fresh fruit) are also encouraged.

1. Greek Meatballs With Tomato Sauce

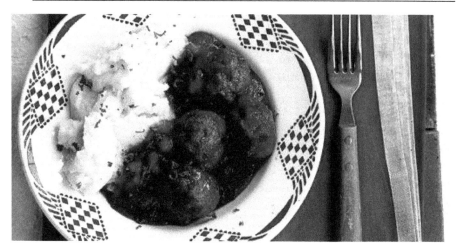

Serves: For 4 People | Ready In 40 Minutes

Nutritional Value

- Calories: 418kcals
- Fat: 21.1g (8.5g Saturated)
- Protein: 29.2g
- Carbohydrates: 24.4g (11.5g Sugars)
- Salt: 1.2g

Ingredients

- 3 thick slices of white bread, crusts removed and torn into pieces
- 125ml red wine
- 500g minced lamb
- 1 small onion, grated

- 1 garlic clove, crushed
- 1 medium egg, beaten
- 1 tbsp chopped fresh parsley, plus extra to garnish
- 1 tsp ground cumin
- 1/2 tsp ground cinnamon

For The Tomato Sauce

- 500ml tomato passata
- 2 tbsp tomato pure
- 2 tbsp tomato ketchup
- 1 tbsp olive oil
- 1 garlic clove, crushed
- 1 tsp sugar
- 1 bay leaf

Method

- Preheat the oven to 180°C/fan160°C/gas 4. Put the bread in a bowl and soak in the wine for 5 minutes. Lightly squeeze out the wine reserving it for the sauce and put the bread pieces into a bowl with the lamb, onion, garlic, egg, parsley, cumin, and cinnamon. Season and mix well.
- Shape the mixture into 12 medium-sized balls, each slightly bigger than a golf ball. Put on a large, non-stick baking sheet and cook for 20 minutes, until golden.

- Meanwhile, combine the reserved wine with all the sauce ingredients in a wide saucepan. Put over medium heat and simmer for 20 minutes, until thickened. Season. Add the meatballs to the sauce and simmer for a further 10 minutes, turning halfway to coat. Discard the bay leaf.
- Divide the meatballs and sauce between serving plates. Serve with mashed potato and garnish with extra parsley.

2. Feta And Pomegranate Salad

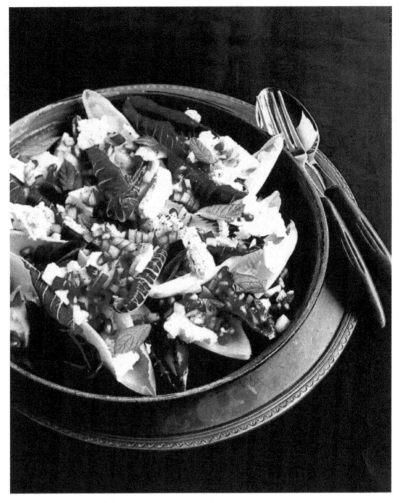

Serves: 4 | Hands-On Time: 15 Mins Plus 30 Mins Resting Time

Nutritional Value

- Calories: 242kcals
- Fat: 18.8g (8.1g Saturated)
- Protein: 9.2g

- Carbohydrates: 10.1g (8g Sugars)
- Salt: 1.8g

Ingredients

- 2 pomegranates, halved
- 1 red onion, finely diced
- 3 tbsp olive oil
- 2 tbsp red wine vinegar
- 200g vegetarian feta
- 2 large chicory heads, 1 red, and 1 white, large leaves roughly torn
- Small bunch of fresh mint, leaves picked

Method

- Working over a bowl, knock out the seeds from each pomegranate half by smacking the skin quite decisively with the back of a wooden spoon. Pick out any strands of pith that escape. Mix the seeds with the onion, oil, and vinegar and season to taste. Set aside for 30 minutes, as the maceration will create a dressing.
- Slice or break the feta into bite-size pieces and add to the pomegranate. Add the chicory to the bowl along with most of the mint leaves, gently combine and transfer to a serving dish. Serve garnished with the remaining mint leaves.

3. Homemade Falafel

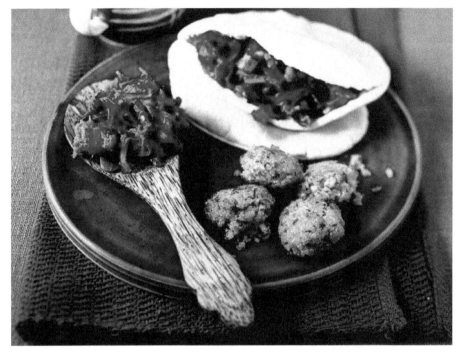

Serves: 4-6 | Takes 1 Hour To Make Plus Soaking Overnight

Nutritional Value

- Calories: 809kcals
- Fat: 28.3g (3.6 Saturated)
- Protein: 29.2g
- Carbohydrates: 116.8g (12.7g Sugar)
- Salt: 4.8g

Ingredients

- 3 tbsp tahini (sesame seed paste, from major supermarkets)
- Juice of 1 lemon
- 200g dried chickpeas, soaked overnight
- 1 level tsp baking powder
- 1 tsp salt
- 2 garlic cloves
- 1 onion, finely diced
- Bunch of fresh coriander, roughly chopped, plus extra to garnish
- Vegetable oil, for frying
- 8-12 pitta bread, warmed and split, to serve

For The Pickle Salad

- 2 small carrots, grated
- ½ small red cabbage, finely sliced
- Juice of ½ lemon
- 2 tbsp extra-virgin olive oil
- 1 tsp salt
- 3 pickled chilies, roughly sliced
- 3 gherkins, roughly sliced

Method

- Make the pickled salad. Mix all the ingredients in a bowl and set aside.
- Make the dressing. Combine the tahini, half the lemon juice, and 50ml water in a bowl. Whisk until smooth, adding a dash of water if its too thick. Season and set aside.
- Drain the chickpeas well, then blitz in a food processor to fine crumbs. Add the remaining lemon juice, baking powder, salt, garlic, onion, and coriander, and blitz again to a pale green pure. Using your hands, shape into 24 small patties.
- Half-fill a large, deep heavy-based saucepan with vegetable oil. Heat until a bread cube turns golden in 1 minute. Fry the fritters, in batches, for 3 minutes, turning once, until golden. Drain on kitchen paper.
- Divide the fritters and salad between the pittas and drizzle with the dressing to serve.

4. Bulgar Wheat, Chickpea And Feta Salad

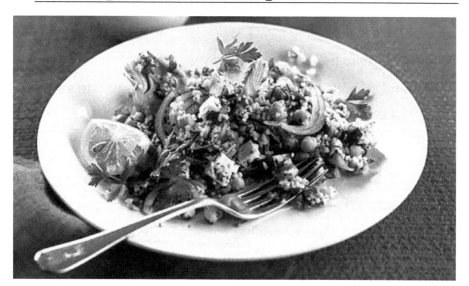

Serves: 6 | Ready In 30 Minutes

Nutritional Value

- Calories: 411
- Protein: 15g
- Fat: 17g
- Carbs: 65g
- Fiber: 15g
- Sugar: 20g

Ingredients

- 75g bulgar wheat
- 25g fresh flatleaf parsley, leaves picked
- and roughly chopped, plus extra whole leaves to garnish
- 1 red onion, finely sliced
- 1 lemon
- 410g can chickpeas, drained and rinsed
- 6 canned artichoke hearts, cut in half
- 150g pack Discover Salad Feta With Red Peppers, drained
- 2 tbsp extra-virgin olive oil

Method

- Rinse the bulgar wheat in cold water. Put in a bowl and cover with hot water. Cover with a cloth and leave for 20 minutes. Drain the bulgar wheat and squeeze out the excess liquid. Stir in the chopped parsley and onion. Cut the lemon in half and squeeze one half over the bulgar wheat, discarding any pips. Cut the other half into wedges and set aside.
- Fold the remaining ingredients into the bulgar wheat. Serve with lemon wedges and a few whole parsley leaves to garnish. You can serve some extra lemon wedges, kalamata olives, and rocket leaves on the side

5. Halloumi And Roasted Veg Kebabs With Basil Spaghetti

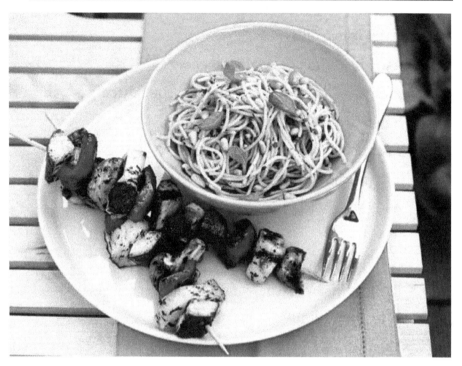

Serves: 4 | Takes 30 Minutes To Make Plus Soaking The Skewers

Nutritional Value

- Calories: 814kcals
- Fat: 45.1g (14.3g Saturated)
- Protein: 27.5g
- Carbohydrates: 85.1g (6.5g Sugar)
- Salt: 1.6g

Ingredients

- 50g fresh basil, plus extra to serve
- 8 tbsp olive oil
- 250g halloumi, drained and cubed
- 1 large red pepper, deseeded and roughly cubed
- 6 mushrooms, halved
- 1 courgette, roughly cubed
- 2 tbsp pine nuts
- 400g spaghetti

Method

- Preheat the barbecue. Soak 8 wooden skewers in water for at least 30 minutes.
- Meanwhile, put the basil, oil, and seasoning in a small food processor or blender and whizz to a pure. Put 2 tablespoons of the mixture into a large bowl. Add the halloumi and vegetables and gently toss them together.
- Meanwhile, heat a frying pan over medium heat. Add the pine nuts and dry-fry for 3-4 minutes, stirring occasionally, until toasted. Set aside. Put a large pan of lightly salted water on to boil, ready for the pasta.
- Thread the halloumi and vegetables alternately onto the skewers. Cook on the hot barbecue for 10 minutes, turning halfway, until the vegetables are just tender.

- Meanwhile, cook the spaghetti according to the packet instructions. Drain well, tip back into the pan, and toss with another 2 tablespoons of the basil mixture and pine nuts. Divide between bowls, scatter with a few basil leaves, and serve with the skewers alongside.

6. Tomato, Egg And Pitta Salad

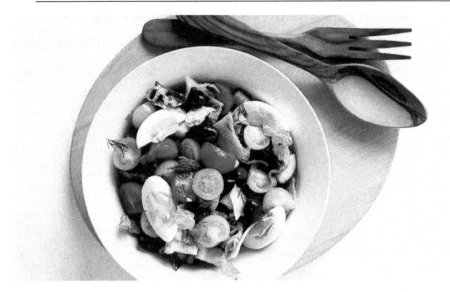

Serves: 4 | Takes 20 Minutes To Make | 6-8 Minutes In The Oven Plus Cooling

Nutritional Value

- Calories: 407kcals
- Fat: 23.7g (4.4g Saturated)
- Protein: 15.1g
- Carbohydrates: 35.6g (6.2g Sugar)
- Salt: 2.2g

Ingredients

- 400g cherry tomatoes, red and yellow, if you like
- 1 cucumber
- 200g purple or green olives, pitted or not, as you prefer

- 3 pitta bread, stale if possible
- 1 small cos lettuce, outer leaves discarded and roughly shredded
- 4 eggs, hard-boiled and cut into wedges
- Small fistful chopped fresh dill
- 2 tbsp red wine vinegar
- 3 tbsp extra-virgin olive oil

Method

- Halve the tomatoes and put them in a large bowl. Deseed the cucumber the easiest way is to halve it lengthways and run the back of a teaspoon along the seed cavity. Dice the cucumber flesh and add it to the bowl along with the olives.
- Preheat the oven to 200°C/fan180°C/gas 6. Split each pitta open and tear it into small pieces. Place on a baking tray and toast in the hot oven for 6-8 minutes, until pale golden and crispy. Cool.
- Divide the lettuce between plates. Toss the cooled, crispy pitta with the tomatoes, cucumber, and olives, and scatter over the lettuce along with the egg and dill. Dress with the vinegar and oil and season to serve.

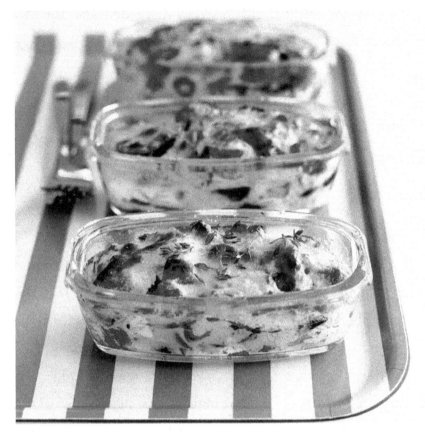

Serves: 6 | Takes 20 Minutes To Make And 45-55 Minutes In The Oven

Nutritional Value

- Calories: 385kcals
- Fat: 22.6g (9.5g Saturated)
- Protein: 18.4g
- Carbohydrates: 28.7g (13.2g Sugar)
- Salt: 2g

Ingredients

- 500g potatoes, cut into chunky slices
- 1 aubergine, sliced
- 1 onion, chopped
- 2 garlic cloves, crushed
- 2 red peppers, deseeded and chopped
- 2 tbsp fresh thyme or marjoram leaves, plus extra leaves to garnish
- 4 tbsp olive oil
- 300g cherry tomatoes
- 250g passata or creamed tomatoes (buy a 500g carton: freeze the rest)
- 250g feta, sliced
- 300ml natural yogurt
- 3 eggs
- 25g vegetarian Parmesan, grated

Method

- Preheat the oven to 230°C/fan210°C/ gas 8. Par-boil the potatoes for 5 minutes, then drain and divide between 2 roasting tins with the aubergine, onion, garlic, and peppers. Sprinkle with the herbs, drizzle with the olive oil, and roast for 20 minutes, turning halfway. Add the tomatoes and cook for 5 minutes, until tender and scorched at the edges. Reduce the oven to 200°C/fan180°C/gas 6.

- Put half the vegetables into 6 x 350ml ovenproof dishes or a 2-liter ovenproof dish. Spoon over half the passata and the feta. Top with the remaining vegetables and passata.
- Mix the yogurt, eggs, and Parmesan in a jug, then pour over the veg. Bake individual dishes for 20 minutes or the large dish for 30 minutes. Check the yogurt mix is firm before serving, garnished with thyme leaves.

8. Pastitsio (Greek pasta bake)

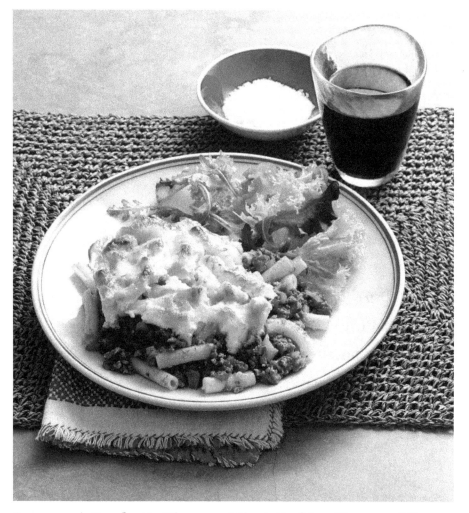

Serves: 4 | Hands-On Time: 45 Mins| Cooking Time: 25 Mins

Nutritional Value

- Calories: 766kcals
- Fat: 31.5g (14.4g Saturated)
- Protein: 44.7g

- Carbohydrates: 80.7g (11.4g Sugars)
- Salt: 0.9g

Ingredients

- 1 tbsp olive oil
- 1 onion, chopped
- 2 garlic cloves, crushed
- 500g lamb mince
- ½ aubergine, chopped
- 2 tbsp tomato pure
- 400g can chopped tomatoes
- 1 tbsp chopped fresh thyme or oregano leaves
- 2 bay leaves
- 150ml hot vegetable stock
- 350g dried macaroni
- 15g butter, softened
- 15g plain flour
- 300ml semi-skimmed or full-fat milk
- 1 egg, lightly beaten
- 50g Cheddar cheese, grated

Method

- Heat the oil in a pan, add the onion and garlic and fry over medium heat for 3 minutes, until softened. Turn the heat to high, add the mince and aubergine and fry for 4 minutes to brown all over. Add the pure, tomatoes, herbs, and stock, bring to the boil, and simmer for 25 minutes until the lamb is tender. Preheat the oven to 180°C/fan160°C/gas 4.

- Meanwhile, cook the macaroni in boiling water according to the packet instructions, then drain and set aside.

- Make the white sauce. Put the butter, flour, and milk into a large jug and whisk. Microwave on high (900W) for 4 minutes, stirring twice until the sauce has boiled and thickened.

- Pour half the macaroni into the base of a 2-liter ovenproof dish, spoon over the meat mixture and top with the rest of the macaroni, or do the same in individual ovenproof dishes. Add the egg to the white sauce, whisk, and pour over the pasta. Sprinkle with the cheese and bake individual pastitsios for 15 minutes or the larger one for 25 minutes, until golden. Serve with a green salad.

9. Minted Lamb And Halloumi Kebabs

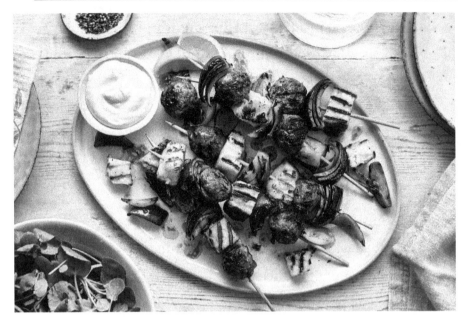

Serves: 6

Hands-On Time: 20 Mins

Cook Time: 10 Mins Plus Marinating

Nutritional Value

- Calories: 468kcals
- Fat: 5.9g (12.2g Saturated)
- Protein: 39g
- Carbohydrates: 19.7g (4.6g Sugars)
- Salt: 2.1g

Ingredients

- 3 tbsp mint sauce
- Juice of 1 small lemon, plus wedges to serve
- 3 tbsp olive oil
- 4 lamb steaks, cubed
- 2 small red onions, 1 cubed, 1 finely sliced
- 1 red pepper, deseeded and cut into squares
- 250g halloumi cheese (from supermarkets), cubed
- 2 x 410g cans mixed pulses, drained, and rinsed
- Small bag of rocket

Method

- Soak 12 bamboo skewers in water for 30 minutes to stop them from burning during cooking. Preheat the grill to high, or light a disposable barbecue.
- Meanwhile, in a bowl, mix the mint sauce, half the lemon juice, and 1 tablespoon oil. Add the lamb, cubed onion, red pepper, and halloumi. Season and mix to coat. Cover and leave for 15 minutes, or chill overnight.
- Put the pulses in a serving bowl with the sliced onion. Add the remaining lemon juice and oil, season, and mix. Set aside, covered.
- Thread the lamb, onion, pepper, and halloumi onto the skewers, being gentle with the halloumi to avoid breaking it. Cook under the hot grill on a baking sheet lined with

foil, or barbecue for 10 minutes, turning halfway until cooked through and lightly charred. Divide between plates. Stir the rocket through the pulses and serve with the kebabs and lemon wedges.

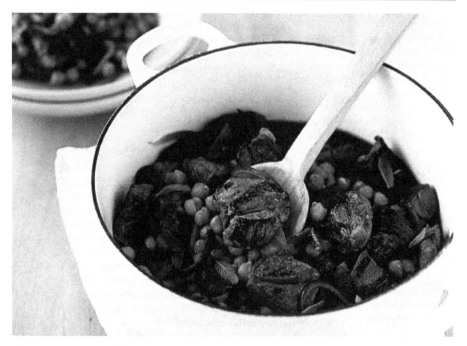

Serves: 4 | Ready In: 40 Minutes

Nutritional Value

Calories: 470kcals | Fat: 20.4g (6.4g Saturated) | Protein: 44.7g | Carbohydrates: 29g (4g Sugars) | Salt: 1.2g

Ingredients

- 1 tbsp vegetable oil
- 650g lamb neck fillets, trimmed of excess fat and cut into cubes (or use lamb leg steaks)
- 2 small red onions, sliced
- ½ tsp ground cumin

- ½ tsp ground coriander
- 2 x 410g cans chickpeas, drained and rinsed
- Juice of 1 lemon
- 300ml fresh vegetable stock, hot
- A small handful of fresh mint leaves, chopped, plus a few extra to garnish

Method

- Heat the oil in a casserole or large, deep saucepan with a lid over high heat. When hot, add half the lamb and cook for 3-4 minutes until browned all over. Remove with a slotted spoon and set aside. Brown the rest of the lamb in the pan, then remove and set aside.
- Reduce the heat to medium. Add the onions to the pan and cook, stirring, for 5 minutes, until softened. Stir in the spices and cook for 1 minute. Add the chickpeas, lemon juice, and stock, plus the lamb and any lamb juices. Mix, cover, and bring to the boil, then reduce to a simmer, covered, for 15 minutes.
- Uncover the casserole and simmer for a further 5 minutes to reduce the sauce slightly. Stir in the mint and season to taste. Divide between 4 shallow bowls and garnish with a few mint leaves.

11. One-Pot Pork, Tomato, And Courgette Rice

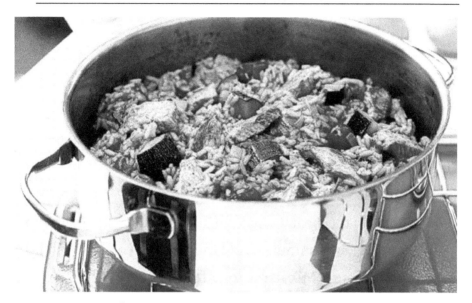

Serves: 4 | Ready In: 45 Minutes

Nutritional Value

- Calories: 541kcals
- Fat: 18.6g (4.2g Saturated)
- Protein: 39.7g
- Carbohydrates: 57g (9.1g Sugars)
- Salt: 1.6g

Ingredients

- 2 tbsp olive oil
- 4 pork loin steaks, fat trimmed, cut into chunks
- 1 onion, chopped

- 200g easy-cook long grain rice
- 1 large courgette, roughly chopped
- 420g jar tomato pasta sauce
- 600ml vegetable stock or water, hot (we like Knorr)

Method

- Put the oil in a deep, non-stick frying pan over high heat. When hot, cook the pork for a few minutes until lightly browned. Remove and set aside.
- Reduce the heat to medium, add the onion, and cook, stirring, for 5 minutes. Add the rice and courgette and stir for 1 minute. Mix in the tomato sauce, stock or water, and pork, plus any juices, and bring to the boil. Reduce the heat and simmer, partially covered, for 30 minutes, stirring occasionally, or until the liquid has been absorbed and the rice is just tender.
- Season to taste and divide between 4 deep plates to serve.

12.Avocados, Prawns, And Mango With Coriander Dressing

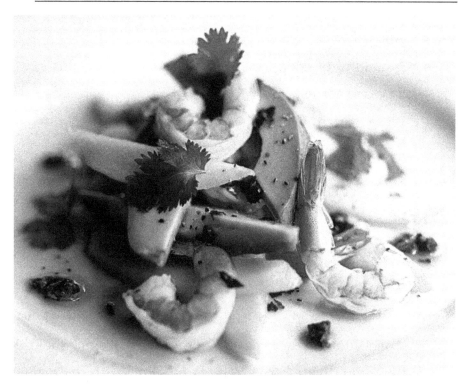

Serves: 4 | Total Time:15 Mins

Nutritional Value

- Calories: 443kcals
- Fat: 37.2g (6.4g Saturated)
- Protein: 18.8g
- Carbohydrates: 8.1g (6.9g Sugars)
- Salt: 3.1g

Ingredients

- 8 tbsp mild olive oil
- Juice of ½ orange
- A handful of chopped fresh coriander leaves, plus extra leaves to garnish
- 1 ripe mango
- 2 ripe avocados
- 300g cooked and peeled large prawns, with tail-shells on

Method

- In a bowl, mix the oil, orange juice, and chopped coriander to make a dressing. Season and set aside.
- Peel, stone, and slice the mango and set aside. Halve, stone, and peel the avocados, discarding the skin. Slice the flesh and divide between 4 plates, along with the mango and prawns. Season to taste.
- Drizzle each plate with the coriander dressing, then scatter with a few coriander leaves to serve.

13. Barbecued Leg Of Lamb With Tomato And Mint Salsa

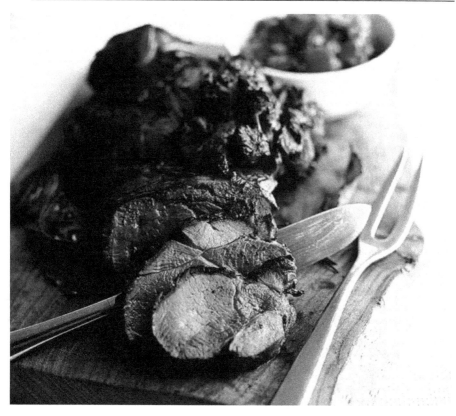

Serves: 6 | Hands-On Time 15 Mins | Cook Time 40-50 Mins Plus Overnight Marinating

Nutritional Value

- Calories: 410kcals
- Fat: 19.1g (0.6g Saturated)
- Protein: 41.6g
- Carbohydrates: 7.6g (6.3g Sugars)
- Salt: Trace

Ingredients

- 1.3-1.5kg leg of lamb, boned and butterflied
- 3 garlic cloves, sliced
- 3 shallots, halved
- Few sprigs of fresh rosemary
- 3 bay leaves
- Few sprigs of fresh oregano
- 375ml red wine
- Vegetable oil, for brushing

For The Tomato And Mint Salsa

- 6 ripe plum or vine tomatoes
- Small bunch of fresh mint, leaves picked
- A good pinch of caster sugar
- Bunch of spring onions, thinly sliced
- 2 garlic cloves, crushed
- 1 tbsp extra-virgin olive oil
- 2 tsp balsamic vinegar

Method

- Put the lamb into a large freezer bag, then add the garlic, shallots, and herbs. Holding the bag carefully, pour in the wine, then seal and put into a container in the fridge. If you have time, leave to marinate for 24 hours or 48 hours for an intense flavor.
- A few hours before you want to eat, make the salsa. Cut the tomatoes in half, scoop out the seeds and discard. Roughly dice the flesh and put it into a bowl. Roughly chop the mint leaves and add to the tomatoes. Sprinkle with the sugar, then add the onions, garlic, olive oil, and balsamic vinegar. Toss well, then set aside to let the flavors develop.
- Take the lamb out of the marinade and discard the marinade. Brush the cooking grate with oil. Barbecue the lamb over direct medium heat for 20-30 minutes, turning once. This will give you medium-cooked meat. If you like your lamb rare, reduce the cooking time by about 5 minutes. Leave to rest for 5 minutes before slicing. Serve with the salsa.

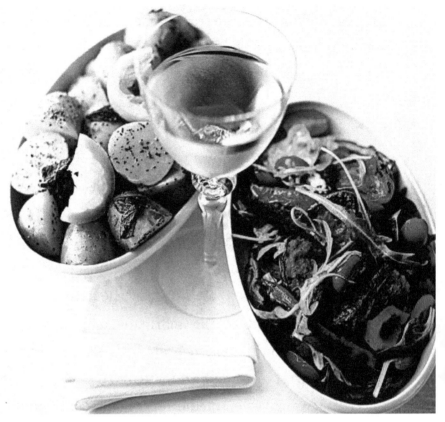

For 6 People | Takes 20 Minutes To Make Plus Cooling

Nutritional Value

- Energy: 205kcals,

- Fats:17.5g (2.5g Saturated),

- Protein: 3.1g

- Carbs: 8.9g

- Sugar: 8.6g

- Salts: 0.1g

Ingredients

- 4 medium courgettes, thickly sliced
- 3 red peppers, halved, deseeded, and cut into wide strips
- Vegetable oil, for tossing
- 2 punnets baby plum tomatoes, halved
- 1 bag rocket leaves
- 1 small bag of baby spinach leaves

For The Dressing

- 6 tbsp extra-virgin olive oil
- 2 tbsp white wine vinegar
- 1/2 tsp Dijon mustard
- Pinch of sugar

Method

- Put the courgettes and peppers into a large bowl and drizzle with a little vegetable oil. Season well and toss to coat. Barbecue over direct heat for 8-10 minutes, turning once (or cook for 8-10 minutes on a hot griddle pan, turning once). Transfer to a large bowl and set aside to cool.
- Meanwhile, make the dressing by whisking all the ingredients together with plenty of seasoning.

- Add the tomatoes, rocket, and spinach to the bowl with the vegetables and toss well. Drizzle with the dressing and toss well again.

15. Sausages With Aubergine Bulgar Pilaf

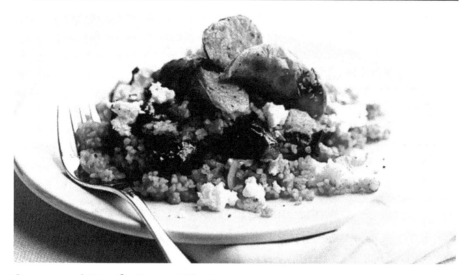

Serves: 4 | Ready In 35 Minutes

Nutritional Value

- Calories: 985kcals
- Fat: 56.2g (19.7g Saturated)
- Protein: 29.2g
- Carbohydrates: 93.5g (9g Sugars)
- Salt: 3.8g

Ingredients

- 6 good-quality pork sausages
- 2 aubergines, cut into large chunks
- 6 tbsp olive oil
- 1 onion, chopped
- 400g bulgur wheat

- 1 tsp ground cinnamon
- 2 tsp tomato pure
- 400g can chopped tomatoes with herbs
- 600ml fresh vegetable stock, hot
- 200g feta, crumbled

Method

- Preheat the oven to 220C/fan200C/gas 7. Put the sausages in one half of a roasting tin, and the aubergines in the other. Drizzle the aubergines with 4 tablespoons of the oil and season. Roast for 25 minutes, turning halfway until cooked through.
- Meanwhile, heat the remaining oil in a large pan over medium heat. Add the onion and cook until softened. Stir in the bulgar wheat, cinnamon, and tomato pure and cook for 1 minute. Add the tomatoes, stock, and season. Cover, reduce the heat, and cook for 15 minutes, stirring occasionally, until the liquid is absorbed. Set aside for 10 minutes, until the bulgar wheat is tender.
- Divide the bulgur wheat and roasted aubergine between plates. Slice the sausages and add them to the plates along with the feta.

16.Cheesy Tuna, Courgette And Spinach Pasta

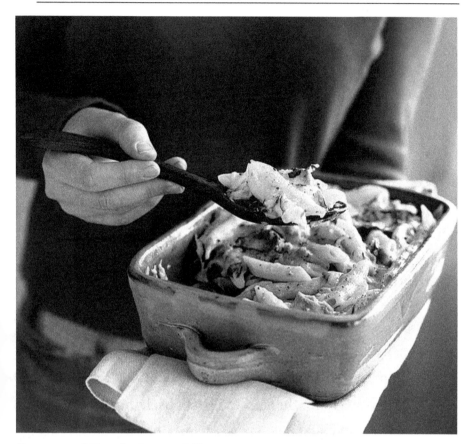

Serves: 4 | Ready In: 20 Minutes

Nutritional Value

- Calories: 559kcals
- Fat: 15.5g (9g Saturated)
- Protein: 34.2g
- Carbohydrates: 74.2g (5.9g Sugars)
- Salt: 0.8g

Ingredients

- 350g penne pasta
- 20g butter, softened
- 20g plain flour
- 250ml semi-skimmed milk
- 100g mature Cheddar, roughly grated
- 1 large courgette, roughly grated
- 2 handfuls spinach leaves, washed and
- large leaves torn
- 200g can tuna steak in spring water, drained

Method

- Bring a large saucepan of salted water to a boil. Add the penne, stir once, bring back to the boil, then simmer for 10 minutes, or cook according to packet instructions, until al dente. Drain, then tip the pasta back into the saucepan.
- Meanwhile, make the cheese sauce. Put the butter in a jug and microwave on high (based on a 900W oven) for 40 seconds, until melted and hot. Stir in the flour to make a paste, then very gradually stir in the milk this will prevent any lumps from forming. Microwave on high for 3-31/2 minutes, stirring every minute until the sauce has thickened. (Alternatively, melt the butter in a pan over medium heat, stir in the flour and cook for 1 minute. Gradually add the milk and cook, stirring, for 6-8 minutes

until the sauce has thickened.) Stir in 60g Cheddar and season to taste.

- Preheat the grill to high. Stir the cheese sauce into the pasta, along with the courgette and spinach, and mix to wilt the spinach. Gently mix in the tuna, then tip into a shallow, 2-liter ovenproof dish. Sprinkle with the remaining cheese. Place directly under the hot grill for 5 minutes, until piping hot and the cheese is turning golden.
- Serve with a green salad.

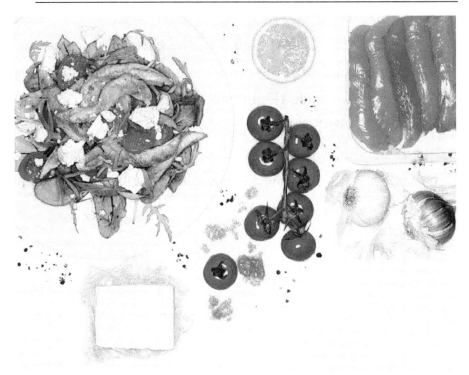

Serves: 3 | Ready In: 20 Minutes

Nutritional Value

- Calories: 540kcals
- Fat: 13.8g (2.1g Saturated)
- Protein: 45.1g
- Carbohydrates: 51.1g (10.5g Sugars)
- Salt: 1g

Ingredients

- 375g pack mini chicken fillets
- Olive oil
- 1 garlic clove, crushed
- 1 small onion, finely sliced
- Punnet cherry tomatoes halved
- Zest of 1 lemon and a squeeze of lemon juice
- Bag of salad
- 150g feta

Method

- Cut the chicken fillets into strips. Heat a little olive oil in a large pan and stir-fry the chicken until tender. Remove and set aside.
- Add the garlic and onion and stir-fry for 2-3 minutes, until softened. Add the cherry tomatoes and stir-fry until beginning to wilt. Add the lemon zest and juice and a good splash of olive oil. Return the chicken to the pan and toss it all together.
- Divide the salad between 3 plates and spoon over the chicken mixture. Crumble the feta between the plates.

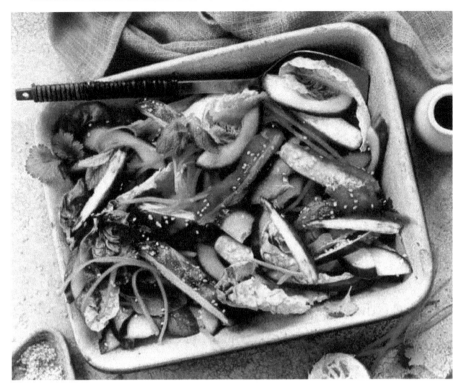

Serves: 4 | Ready In: 20 Minutes

Nutritional Value

- Calories: 291kcals
- Fat: 11.5g (1.8g Saturated)
- Protein: 30.2g
- Carbohydrates: 16.2g (15.2g Sugars)
- Fibre: 4.3g
- Salt: 3G

Ingredients

- 3 free-range skinless chicken breasts
- 3 tbsp soy sauce
- 2 tbsp honey
- 2 tbsp toasted sesame oil
- 1 cucumber, deseeded and sliced into half-moons
- 4 carrots, sliced into fine strips
- Large handful each of fresh coriander and fresh mint leaves picked
- 4 little gem lettuces, torn
- 1 tbsp groundnut or vegetable oil
- Juice of 2 limes
- 1 tbsp fish sauce
- Sesame seeds to serve

Method

- Put the chicken between two pieces of cling film, then flatten with a meat mallet or rolling pin until 1-1.5cm thick. Put the chicken in a shallow dish with soy, honey, and 1 tbsp of sesame oil. Leave for 10 minutes.
- Meanwhile, prepare the salad. Put the cucumber, carrots, herbs, and lettuces in a large serving bowl or on a platter, then set aside.
- Heat the groundnut/vegetable oil in a frying pan over high heat, then fry the marinated chicken for 2 minutes on each

side until cooked through and glazed. Remove from the heat, cool a little, then slice into strips.

- In a small bowl or jug, mix the lime juice, fish sauce, and remaining sesame oil. Add the chicken and dressing to the salad and toss to combine, then sprinkle with sesame seeds and serve.

19.Roast Pepper And Garlic Salad With Hazelnuts

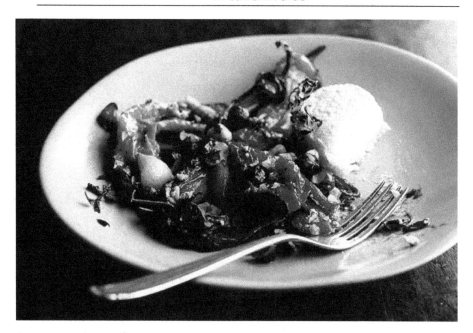

Serves: 4 | Ready In: 1 Hour

Nutritional Value

- Calories: 304kcals
- Fat: 24.8g (2.3g Saturated)
- Protein: 6.7g
- Carbohydrates: 15g (11.3g Sugar)
- Salt: 1.3g

Ingredients

- 2 large red peppers
- 2 large yellow peppers

- 1 fat garlic bulb, cloves whole and unpeeled
- 3 tbsp olive oil
- 1 tsp salt
- Small bunch oregano or marjoram, leaves picked
- 1 tbsp sherry or balsamic vinegar
- 100g whole hazelnuts

Method

- Preheat the oven to 200°C/fan180°C/gas 6. Cut the peppers lengthways into rough quarters, discarding any seeds and pith, but leaving the stalks on. Lay them on baking trays skin-side up. Scatter the peppers with garlic, olive oil, salt, oregano, and sherry or balsamic vinegar, and cover with foil. Roast for 20 minutes. Remove the foil and return to the oven for another 15 minutes, or until wilted their skins should be brown and wrinkly. (Leave the oven on to roast the nuts.) Set aside for at least 15 minutes.
- Meanwhile, spread the hazelnuts in a single layer on a baking sheet and cook in the oven for 5 minutes until golden. Remove and cool slightly, then roughly crush in a pestle and mortar. Transfer the peppers, garlic, and juices to a serving bowl, then scatter the lightly crushed nuts over the top. Squeeze the garlic out of its skin with your fingers as you eat the salad.

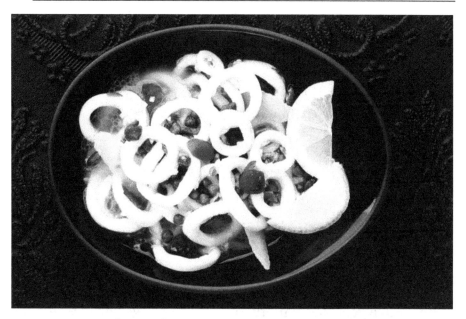

Serves: 4 People | Takes :25 Minutes To Make Plus Overnight Marinating

Nutritional Value

- Calories: 305kcals
- Fat: 22.4g (3.4g Saturated)
- Protein: 23.7g
- Carbohydrates: 4g (0.7g Sugar)
- Salt: 0.8g

Ingredients

- 600g squid, cleaned, gutted, and cut into rings
- Juice of 3 unwaxed lemons, with their leaves if possible
- 2 tbsp capers
- 3 garlic cloves, finely sliced
- Few whole black peppercorns
- Handful pitted Kalamata, halved, or whole small black olives
- 100ml extra-virgin olive oil

Method

- Put a generous handful of salt into a large pan of water and bring to a rolling boil. Blanch the squid in the pan for no more than 30 seconds, then drain. Alternatively, sear it on a ridged griddle or cast-iron frying pan for about 30 seconds on either side.
- Using a potato peeler or fruit knife, peel 4 or 5 strips of lemon zest and put them in a mixing bowl. If the lemons have leaves, de-stalk and shred two of them to add to the zest. (You could use bay leaves instead.)
- Add the capers to the bowl after soaking and rinsing them if they are packed in salt. Add the lemon juice, garlic, peppercorns, olives, and oil. Mix thoroughly, then stir in the squid while still warm. Cover and marinate in the fridge, ideally overnight.

- Serve with lemon wedges. This is great with thin slices of fennel or chicory, or pop it on toast or toss with warm new potatoes. It shouldnt need salt but check to make sure.

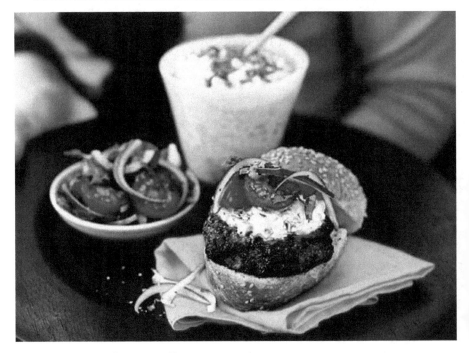

Serves: 4 People | Ready In: 30 Minutes

Nutritional Value

- Calories: 323kcals
- Fat: 2.3g (0.4g Saturated)
- Protein: 37.7g
- Carbohydrates: 39.8g (8.5g Sugar)
- Salt: 1.8g

Ingredients

- 1 large red onion
- 12 cherry tomatoes, halved

- Large handful chopped fresh coriander
- 450g turkey mince or you can use lean chicken, lamb, or pork mince
- 2 tbsp sweet chili dipping sauce
- 1 tbsp soy sauce
- 1/4 cucumber
- 150g carton 0% fat greek yogurt
- Small handful chopped fresh mint
- Tabasco sauce, to taste
- 4 crusty burger buns, toasted

Method

- Thinly slice a quarter of the onion and mix with the tomatoes and half the coriander. Season and set aside.
- Coarsely grate the remaining onion and mix well with the turkey mince, sweet chili sauce, soy sauce, remaining coriander, and plenty of black pepper. Form into 4 burgers, which are slightly larger than the burger buns. (The mixture will be quite wet, but, when cooked, will give you moist, juicy burgers.)
- Preheat the grill to hot. Arrange the burgers on a foil-lined grill pan and grill for 6 minutes on each side.
- Meanwhile, halve the cucumber lengthways, scoop out the seeds with a teaspoon and discard. Dice and mix with the yogurt, mint, seasoning, and Tabasco.

- Grill the burger buns until toasted. Arrange a burger on each toasted bun base, top with a spoonful of tzatziki, then tomato salad, and finally, the burger tops to serve.

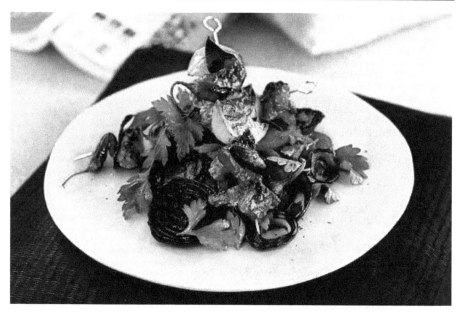

Serves: 4 People | Takes: 50 Minutes To Make Plus Marinating

Nutritional Value

- Calories: 246kcals
- Fat: 8.7g (2.2g Saturated)
- Protein: 29g
- Carbohydrates: 14.4g (10.1g Sugar)
- Salt: 0.3g

Ingredients

- 3 small lemons
- 500g pork fillet (tenderloin), trimmed of all fat and cut into 32 small pieces

- 4 garlic cloves, crushed
- 1 tsp dried oregano
- 1 tsp each ground cumin, coriander, and turmeric
- 2 tsp paprika
- 4 tbsp 0% fat Greek yogurt
- 16 fresh bay leaves
- 16 whole pickled red chilies (optional)
- 3 red onions, thickly sliced
- 3 beef tomatoes, thickly sliced
- 1 tbsp olive oil
- Balsamic vinegar, for drizzling
- A large handful tore fresh flatleaf parsley

Method

- Finely grate the zest from 1 lemon and squeeze the juice. Put both into a bowl with the pork, garlic, oregano, ground spices, and yogurt. Mix well, cover, and set aside to marinate for at least 20 minutes (or up to 2 hours if you have the time).
- Preheat the grill to hot. Cut each of the remaining lemons into 8 wedges. Thread 4 pieces of pork, 2 wedges of lemon, 2 bay leaves, and 2 chilies alternately on each skewer. Arrange on a large foil-lined grill tray and grill for 15 minutes, turning, until the pork is cooked through and lightly charred.

- Meanwhile, preheat the oven to 180°C/fan160°C/ gas 4, and heat a large griddle pan until smoking. Brush the onions and tomatoes with the oil and season well. Chargrill the onions for 5 minutes, turn them over, and cook for a further 2 minutes.

- Transfer to a baking dish and keep hot in the oven while you cook the tomatoes. Add the tomatoes to the griddle pan and chargrill for 2-3 minutes, without turning.

- Pile the tomatoes onto serving plates with the onions and sprinkle over some balsamic vinegar and flatleaf parsley. Arrange the spiced pork skewers on top to serve.

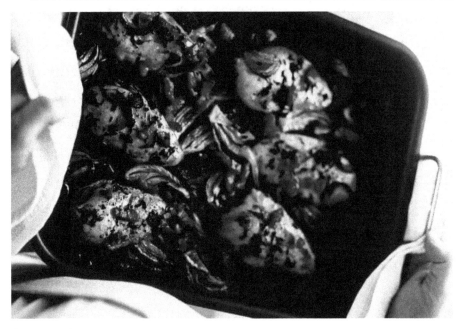

Serves: 6

Nutrition Value

- Calories: 371kcals
- Fat: 17.7g (5g Saturated)
- Protein: 41.6g
- Carbohydrates: 3g (2.2g Sugars)
- Salt: 1.9g

Ingredients

- 4 tbsp olive oil
- 4 garlic cloves, finely sliced
- 20g bunch fresh thyme, leaves picked
- 6 boneless, skinless chicken breasts
- 200g smoked lardons or pancetta pieces
- 2 fennel bulbs, each cut into 12 wedges
- 1 red onion, sliced into 12 wedges
- 300ml dry white wine

Method

- Preheat the oven to 200°C/fan180°C/gas 6. Put 2 tablespoons of the oil into a non-stick roasting tin. Add the garlic, thyme, 1 tablespoon sea salt and 2 teaspoons ground black pepper and mix. Add the chicken and turn to coat. Scatter with the lardons or pancetta, add the fennel and onion, and drizzle with the remaining oil. Cook for 15 minutes, then increase the oven temperature to 230°C/fan210°C/gas 8.
- Pour the wine into the tin and cook for another 10 minutes, or until the chicken is golden and the vegetables tender. Serve with the Lemon-dressed tagliatelle

24.   Roast Pork Steaks With Tomatoes And Pine Nuts

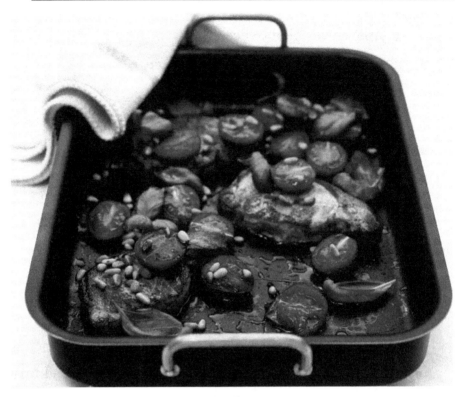

Serves: 4 | Ready In: 30 Minutes

Nutritional Value

- Calories: 462kcals
- Fat: 31.7g (10g Saturated)
- Protein: 40.2g
- Carbohydrates: 4g (4.2g Sugar)
- Salt: 0.3g

Ingredients

- 1 tbsp olive oil, plus extra for drizzling
- 4 pork loin steaks or chops
- 250g vine-ripened midi plum tomatoes
- 25g pine nuts
- Good splash balsamic vinegar
- Large bunch basil

Method

- Preheat the oven to 180°C/fan160°C/gas 4. Heat the olive oil in a large pan and cook the pork steaks or chops for 1-2 minutes each side until golden brown. Transfer to a large roasting tin spaced well apart. Cut the tomatoes in half and scatter over the pork, followed by the pine nuts. Season well. Put the roasting tray in the oven and roast for 12-15 minutes until the pork is tender.
- Remove from the oven, sprinkle over the vinegar and scatter with the fresh basil leaves. Spoon the pork, tomatoes, and basil on 4 warm plates. Serve drizzled with a little extra olive oil.

25.   Salmon With Basil, Lemon And Olive Butter

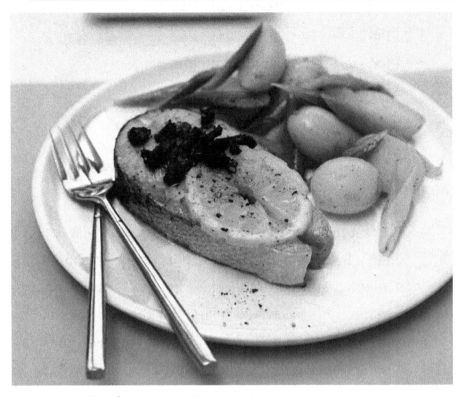

Serves: 4 | Ready In: 20 Minutes

Nutritional Value

- Calories: 417kcals
- Fat: 29.9g (10.4g Saturated)
- Protein: 35.9g
- Carbohydrates: 1g (0.6g Sugar)
- Salt: 0.6g

Ingredients

- Large handful of fresh basil
- 1 large lemon
- 4 pitted black olives, roughly chopped
- 50g butter, softened
- 4 salmon steaks, about 175g each
- Cooked new potatoes, to serve
- Sliced leeks, to serve

Method

- Preheat the oven to 200°C/fan180°C/gas 6. Roughly chop the basil and put it into a large bowl. Grate the zest of 1/2 lemons and add to the bowl with the black olives. Add the butter and beat well with a wooden spoon until mixed. Put aside.

- Put the salmon steaks into an ovenproof dish large enough to fit the salmon in a single layer. Score the zest of the remaining 1/2 lemons with a canceled knife. You dont have to do this but it looks pretty. Cut 4 slices from the half of lemon you have just canelled and place one on top of each steak. Divide the olive butter into 4 and spoon on top of each lemon slice. Cover the dish with foil and bake in the oven for 12 minutes until just tender.

- Divide the salmon between plates and spoon over the melted butter. Season and serve with cooked new potatoes and steamed and sliced baby leeks.

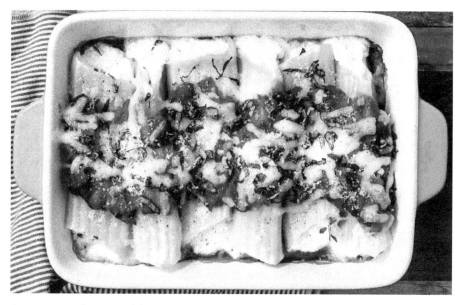

Serves: 4 | Prep Time: 10 Minutes | Cook Time: 30 Minutes | Total Time: 40 Minutes

Ingredients

- 1/2 cup onions
- 4 cloves garlic
- 1 batch vegan ricotta from my Vegan Ricotta Zucchini Casserole, prepared
- 8 Manicotti shells (I used gluten-free)
- 1 15 oz tomato sauce
- salt, pepper to taste
- 1 batch Vegan Parmesan Cheese (3 ingredients, 1 min), prepared

Instructions

- While you pre-cook your shells, prepare the filling. In a pan heat a bit of oil, or vegetable broth, and add garlic and onions. Fry this mix for around 3 minutes, then adds optional mushrooms before frying for 2 minutes longer.
- Also, the last-minute adds optional spinach to that pan. Take it from the stove and mix everything in the pan with the vegan ricotta and half of the prepared vegan Parmesan. Reserve the rest for the topping, and season with salt and pepper.
- Set all aside, and preheat oven to 415°F. You will need an 8x11 inch casserole dish. Start with a layer of tomato sauce, so the bottom of your baking dish is covered.
- Now use the Manicotti filling and give about 3 tsp into the noodles. Place them in the oven dish, repeat that until all shells are stuffed. Give the rest of the filling on top, cover everything with the remaining marinara and the reserved vegan Parmesan.
- Bake all for 30 minutes, then divide on to plates.

Nutrition Information

- Calories: 324| Total Fat: 10.4g| Saturated Fat: 5.4g| Trans Fat: 0g| Unsaturated Fat: 3.7g| Cholesterol: 0mg| Sodium: 63mg| Carbohydrates: 40.2g| Fiber: 3.5g| Sugar: 7.5g |Protein: 16.7g

27.Spanish Rice and Beans

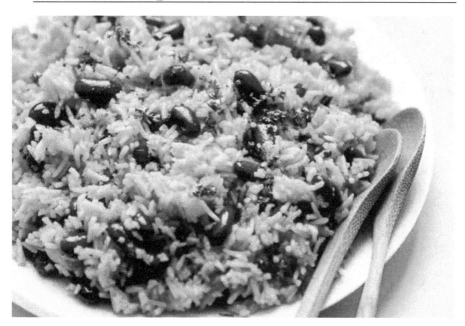

Yield: 4 | Prep Time: 5 Minutes | Cook Time: 12 Minutes | Total Time: 17 Minutes

Ingredients

- 1 cup cooked black beans
- 5 cloves garlic
- 2 cups uncooked rice
- 2 cups tomato sauce
- 1 cup vegetable broth
- 4 tsp smoked paprika
- Salt, pepper to taste

Instructions

- Heat a pot with a bit of oil - or vegetable broth if you avoid oil. Add minced garlic, optional bell pepper, and onions.
- Fry everything for around 3 minutes before adding uncooked rice, tomato sauce, vegetable broth, smoked paprika, and optional soaked saffron.
- Cook everything according to the rice package instructions. Mine was ready in 8 minutes, so it depends on your rice and brand. Last mix in optional olives and parsley.
- Serve on plates or bowls and devour, yum.

Nutrition Information

Calories: 198| Total Fat: 0.8g| Saturated Fat: 0.2g| Trans Fat: 0g| Unsaturated Fat: 0.4g| Cholesterol: 0mg| Sodium: 140mg| Carbohydrates: 41g| Fiber: 6g| Sugar: 4.8g| Protein: 7.7g

28.   Cajun Pasta

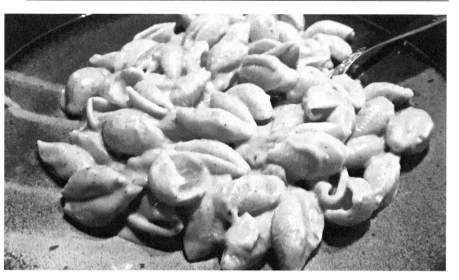

Yield: 6 | Prep Time: 5 Minutes | Cook Time: 10 Minutes | Total Time: 15 Minutes

Ingredients

- 10 Oz Pasta (Use Gluten-Free If Needed)
- 1 15 Oz Can Chopped Tomatoes
- 2 Tbsp Cajun Seasoning
- 1/2 Cup Coconut Milk
- 5 Cloves Garlic
- 1 Cup Cooked Black Beans
- Salt, Pepper To taste

Instructions

- First cook your favorite pasta according to the package directions. The actual time will vary a bit depending on your used pasta shapes. While pasta is cooking heat a pan or pot with a bit of oil, vegan butter, or just vegetable broth for oil-free cooking.
- Start with optional onions, bell peppers, minced garlic, and fry all for 3 minutes. After that add optional sliced mushrooms.
- Finally, make the cajun pasta sauce. Just add chopped tomatoes, black beans, and coconut milk to the same pan. Season with cajun seasoning, salt, pepper, and again optional smoked paprika if you like. Cook for an additional 5 minutes, drain pasta and mix with cajun sauce. Serve on a plate or in bowls, enjoy.

Nutrition Information

- Calories: 359| Total Fat: 5.8g| Saturated Fat: 4.4g| Unsaturated Fat: 0.5g| Csodium: 640mg| Carbohydrates: 70.5g| Fiber: 12.2g| Sugar: 4.7g| Protein: 18.7g

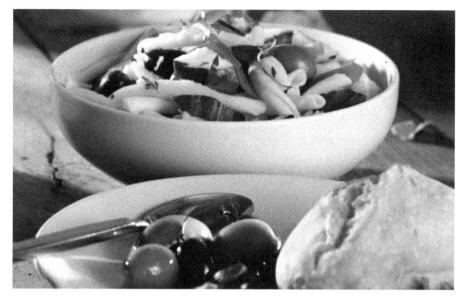

Yield: 4 | Prep Time: 10 Minutes | Total Time: 10 Minutes

Ingredients

For The Salad:

- 4 cups pasta cooked (use of, f needed)
- 1/2 cup red onions, finely chopped
- 1/2 cup cherry tomatoes, halved
- 1 cup bell pepper (i used yellow) finely chopped
- 1/3 cup cucumber finely chopped
- 1 cup olives (kalamata are great) halved and pitted
- 1 cup vegan feta, finely chopped
- Salt, pepper to taste

For The Dressing:

- 1/4 cup olive oil
- 1/4 cup red vinegar
- 3 cloves garlic, pressed
- 2 tsp dill, dried
- 2 tsp oregano, dried
- Salt, pepper to taste

Instructions

- Start with a small bowl. Combine garlic, dill, oregano, red vinegar, olive oil, and season with salt and pepper. Mix it all until combined. Set the dressing aside.
- Next, in a larger bowl, combine pasta, cucumber, tomatoes, onions, bell pepper, vegan feta, and olives. Add dressing and mix. Serve on plates or in bowls.

Nutrition Information

- Calories: 515| Total Fat: 14g| Saturated Fat: 8g| Trans Fat: 0g| Unsaturated Fat: 4g| Cholesterol: 0mg| Sodium: 301mg| Carbohydrates: 54g| Fiber: 4g| Sugar: 0.7g| Protein: 11g

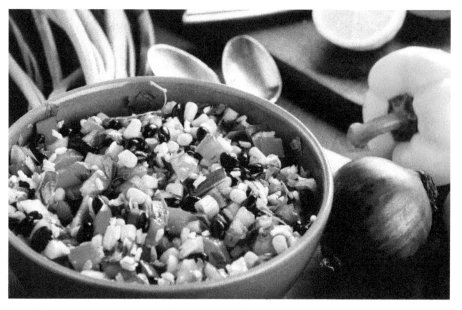

Yield: 4 | Prep Time: 5 Minutes | Cook Time: 12 Minutes | Total
Time: 17 Minutes

Ingredients

- 1 cup quinoa, uncooked
- 1 1/2 cups black beans, cooked
- 1 cup black-eyed peas, cooked
- 1/2 cup corn
- 5 cloves garlic minced
- 1/3 cup italian dressing
- Salt, pepper to taste

Instructions

- First cook your quinoa according to package directions. You will need to wash and drain it.
- While the quinoa is cooking, prepare the salad: drain cooked beans, corn, and mix with cooked quinoa.
- Finally: make the dressing by combining the Italian dressing with minced garlic and the optional spices such as cumin, chili powder, and orange juice.
- Toss in the salad and divide between plates or bowls.

Nutrition Information

- Calories: 446| Total Fat: 6g| Saturated Fat: 1g| Trans Fat: 0g| Unsaturated Fat: 1g| Cholesterol: 0mg| Sodium: 930mg| Carbohydrates: 74g| Fiber: 21g| Sugar: 2.5g| Protein: 23g

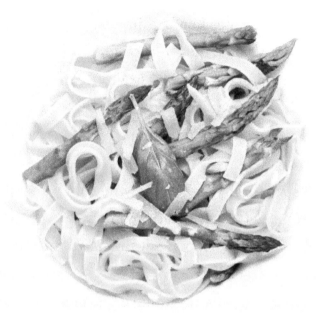

Yield: 2 | Prep Time: 3 Minutes | Cook Time: 10 Minutes | Total Time: 13 Minutes

Ingredients

- 8 oz pasta (use gf, if needed)
- 1 tbsp olive oil
- 7 oz green asparagus tips
- 8 oz soy cuisine
- 1 tbsp garlic powder
- 1 tbsp onion powder
- 6 oz vegan chicken cubes
- Salt, pepper to taste

Instructions

- Bring salted water to a boil in a large pot and cook your pasta according to the directions.
- While the pasta is cooking, heat olive oil in a pan. When hot, add the vegan chicken strips, season them with salt and pepper and fry for around 3 minutes until slightly browned.
- Add asparagus tip and fry everything for 3 minutes longer. Add soy cuisine, garlic, and onion and season with another pinch of salt and pepper. Let simmer on medium heat for an extra 5 minutes.
- When the pasta is ready, drain it and mix it with asparagus sauce in the saucepan.

Nutrition Information

- Calories: 680| Total Fat: 30.8g| Saturated Fat: 9g| Trans Fat: 0g| Unsaturated Fat: 12.4g| Cholesterol: 0mg| Sodium: 543mg| Carbohydrates: 58.9g| Fiber: 24.4g| Sugar: 5.6g| Protein: 70.2g

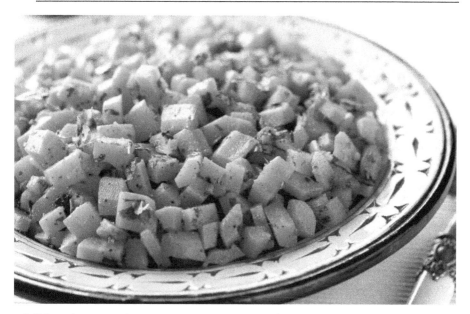

Yield: 6 | Prep Time: 10 Minutes | Cook Time: 15 Minutes | Total Time: 25 Minutes

Ingredients

- 1 lb carrots, shredded
- 1 cup raisins
- 3/4 cup pistachios, peeled and chopped
- 1 15 oz can chickpeas
- salt, pepper to taste
- 30 Seconds Best Hummus Recipe
- Ras El Hanout Spice blend (1/2 tsp turmeric, 2 tsp cumin, 1 tsp paprika, 1/2 tsp cinnamon, 1/4 tsp ground cloves)

Instructions

- In a bowl, combine drained chickpeas, Ras El Hanout spice blend. Take 1/3 cup from your prepared hummus and mix with everything. On a baking sheet prepared with parchment paper, bake the chickpeas for around 15 minutes at 410°F.
- Assembling the salad: mix shredded carrots, raisins, pistachios, roasted chickpeas in a bowl. Top with the remaining hummus. Divide into plates or devour straight from the bowl.

Nutrition Information

- Calories: 280| Total Fat: 10g| Saturated Fat: 1g| Trans Fat: 0g| Unsaturated Fat: 1g| Cholesterol: 0mg| Sodium: 302mg| Carbohydrates: 46g| Fiber: 9g| Sugar: 19g| Protein: 9g

33.   10 Minute Mediterranean Vegan Pasta

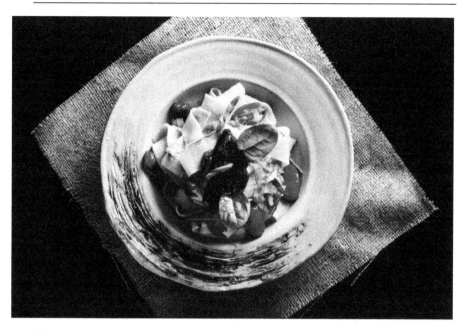

Yield: 6 | Cook Time: 10 Minutes | Total Time: 10 Minutes

Ingredients

- 10 oz of your favorite pasta (I used gluten-free)
- 1 cup hummus
- 1/3 cup water
- 5 cloves garlic, minced or pressed
- 1/2 cup olives
- 1/2 cup walnuts
- 2 Tbs dried cranberries, optional
- Salt, pepper to taste

Instructions

- Cook the pasta according to the manufacturer's directions.
- While the pasta is cooking prepare the hummus sauce: combine hummus, water, and garlic, then season with salt and pepper. Finally add olives, walnuts, and optional dried cranberries. When the pasta is done, drain, and combine with the sauce.

Nutrition Information

- Calories: 620| Total Fat: 12g| Saturated Fat: 6g| Trans Fat: 0g| Unsaturated Fat: 4g| Cholesterol: 0mg| Sodium: 250mg| Carbohydrates: 79g| Fiber: 1g| Sugar: 1g| Protein: 26g

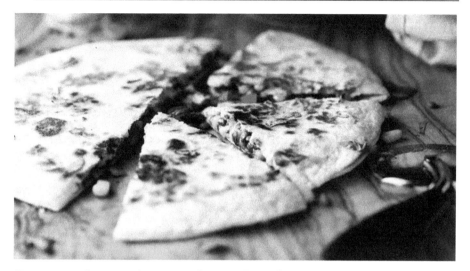

Serves: 12 | Prep Time: 5 Minutes | Cook Time: 15 Minutes | Total Time: 20 Minutes

Ingredients

For The Vegan Cheese

- 1 can corn
- 4 tbs nutritional yeast
- 5 cloves garlic
- Salt, pepper

For The Quesadillas

- 1-2 smashed avocado
- 1 cup cherry tomatoes
- Your favorite tortillas (i used gluten-free flour tortillas)

- Optional chill powder for a bit more heat

Instructions

Prepare The Vegan Cheese:

- Combine corn, garlic, nutritional yeast, salt, and pepper to taste in the bowl of a blender or food processor. process until the mixture is well combined. Dont over-process or it will end up too smooth.

Make The Quesadillas:

- Put smashed avocado on your favorite tortilla. Add cherry tomatoes, cut in halves. Top all of it with a really good amount of vegan cheese. If you like, add a bit more heat with the optional chill powder. Finish with the second tortilla.
- Cut the quesadilla into triangles, brush them with a bit of oil if needed. Bake at 400Â°F on a baking sheet with parchment paper for around 15 minutes until crispy and golden.

Nutrition Information

Calories: 189| Total Fat: 12g| Saturated Fat: 6g| Trans Fat: 0g| Unsaturated Fat: 4g| Cholesterol: 0mg| Sodium: 360mg| Carbohydrates: 12g| Fiber: 1g| Sugar: 1.1g| Protein: 8g

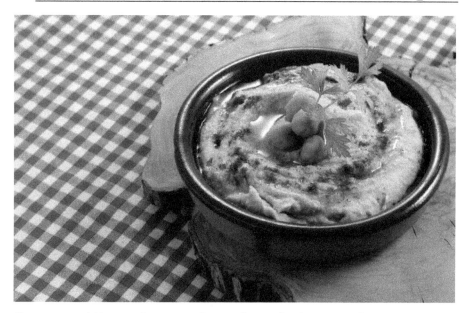

Serves: 12 | Prep Time: 1 Minute | Total Time: 1 Minute

Ingredients

- 1 15 oz can chickpeas + brine (do not drain use the brine)
- 1/3 cup water
- 5 cloves garlic
- 2 tsp cumin
- Juice of 1 lemon
- 3/4 cup Tahini
- salt, pepper

Instructions

- Combine all the ingredients in the bowl of a high-speed blender. Start with the liquid, followed by chickpeas with the brine and then all the other ingredients. Use the manual setting and the highest speed and use a tamper. Process until smooth, after 30 seconds, done.

Nutrition Information

- Calories: 100| Total Fat: 5g| Saturated Fat: 1g| Trans Fat: 0g| Unsaturated Fat: 4g| Cholesterol: 0mg| Sodium: 227mg| Carbohydrates: 8g| Fiber: 3g| Sugar: 0g| Protein: 5g

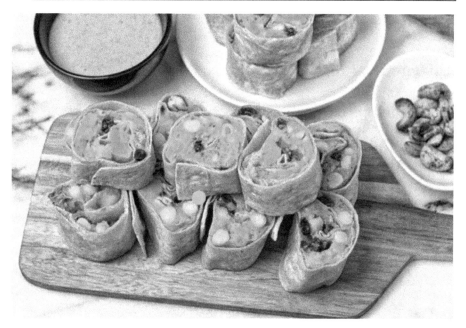

Yield: 24 | Cook Time: 10 Minutes | Total Time: 10 Minutes

Ingredients

- 2 sweet potatoes, peeled and cut into cubes.
- 1 15 oz can chickpeas
- 1/2 cup coconut oil at room temperature
- 5 cloves garlic, peeled and pressed
- Salt, pepper to taste

Thai Green Curry Sauce

- 4 tortillas, gluten-free

Instructions

- First cook the sweet potatoes in a steamer in the microwave for about 8 minutes until they are soft. Alternatively, just cook them, then mash them with coconut oil and chickpeas. Use a potato masher or fork, then mix with garlic, salt, and pepper.
- Assemble your pinwheels: put 2 heaping Tbs of the potato mixture in your tortillas, sprinkle with Thai Green Curry sauce, roll.

Nutrition Information

- Calories: 100| Total Fat: 6.3g| Saturated Fat: 1.5g| Trans Fat: 0g| Unsaturated Fat: 4.1g| Cholesterol: 0mg| Sodium: 87mg| Carbohydrates: 7.1g| Fiber: 0.7g| Sugar: 0.2g| Protein: 2.8g

37.Garlic Noodles Recipe

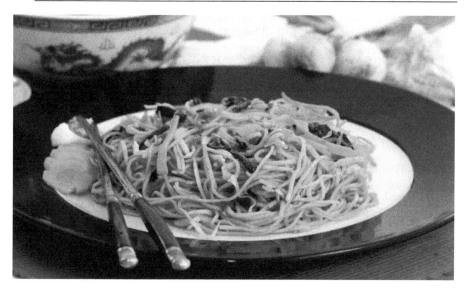

Serves: 6 | Prep Time: 3 Minutes | Cook Time: 12 Minutes | Total Time: 15 Minutes

Ingredients

- 1 lb pasta (use gluten-free, if needed)
- 6 tbs vegan butter
- 10 cloves garlic, minced
- 1 batch vegan parmesan cheese (3 ingredients, 1 min), prepared
- 1 tbs coconut milk
- Salt, pepper to taste

Instructions

- First cook your pasta according to the package directions.
- While you do this, heat a pot and bring the vegan butter to melt, and add minced garlic. Fry it for around 4 minutes on low to medium heat. Stir in the vegan Parmesan and coconut milk until everything is well combined.
- By now the pasta should be done. Drain, then give to the pot with the creamy garlic sauce. Mix well with and cook all over medium heat for 2 minutes. Finally, season with salt and pepper and serve on plates or in bowls.

Nutrition Information

- Calories: 498| Total Fat: 20.7g| Saturated Fat: 11.9g| Trans Fat: 0g| Unsaturated Fat: 2.8g| Cholesterol: 0mg| Sodium: 75mg| Carbohydrates: 63.9g| Fiber: 3.2g| Sugar: 2.1g| Protein: 12.6g

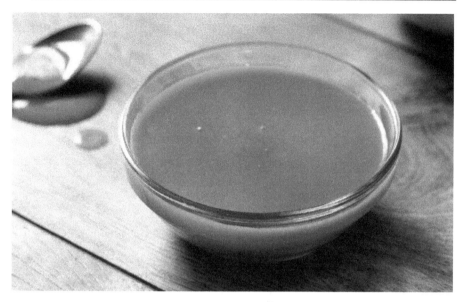

Serves: 12 | Prep Time: 5 Minutes | Cook Time: 5 Minutes | Total Time: 10 Minutes

Ingredients

- 1/2 cup vegan butter
- 3/4 cup hot sauce
- 2 cloves garlic minced
- 3 tsp maple syrup
- 1/4 cup white vinegar
- Salt, pepper to taste

Instructions

- Heat vegan butter in a pot, then add minced garlic, maple syrup, hot sauce, and vinegar.
- Add a pinch of salt and pepper and heat everything until it simmers. Turn down the heat to make sure not to overcook and let it simmer for around 5 minutes.
- Let the sauce cool completely, then store in an airtight container or sealed jar.

Nutrition Information

- Calories: 68| Total Fat: 6.7g| Saturated Fat: 5.3g| Trans Fat: 0g| Unsaturated Fat: 0.1g| Cholesterol: 0mg| Sodium: 40mg| Carbohydrates: 0.7g| Fiber: 0.1g| Sugar: 1.1g| Protein: 0.1g

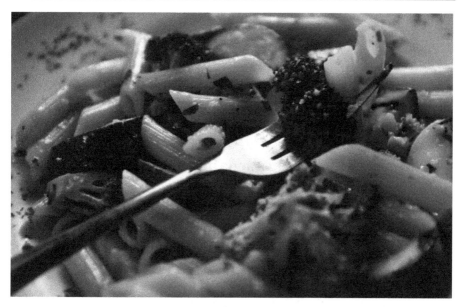

Serves: 2 | Prep Time: 2 Minutes | Cook Time: 8 Minutes | Total Time: 10 Minutes

Ingredients

- 1 cup white wine
- 5 cloves garlic
- 7 oz oat cream
- 2 tsp garlic powder
- 2 tbsp nutritional yeast
- Salt, pepper to taste

Instructions

- First, in a saucepan, heat a bit of oil, vegan butter, or vegetable broth if you are into oil-free cooking. Now add minced garlic and fry for around 3 minutes.
- Slowly add oat cream, white wine, nutritional yeast, garlic powder, and season with salt and pepper. Cook everything for around 5 minutes and you are done.

Nutrition Information

- Calories: 280| Total Fat: 12.8g| Saturated Fat: 1g| Trans Fat: 0g| Unsaturated Fat: 10g| Cholesterol: 0mg| Sodium: 7.5mg| Carbohydrates: 13g| Fiber: 2.7g| Sugar: 4.6g| Protein: 4.6g

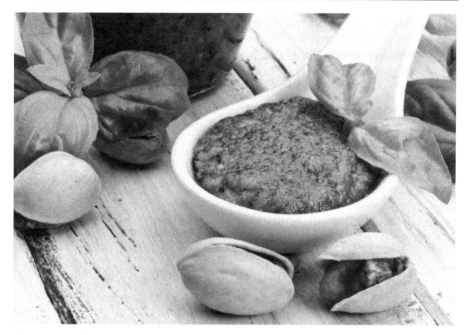

Serves: 8 | Prep Time: 3 Minutes | Total Time: 3 Minutes

Ingredients

- 1/2 cup pistachios
- 1 cup basil
- 5 cloves garlic
- 1 cup olive oil
- 3/4 cup Vegan Parmesan Cheese (3 ingredients, 1 min), prepared

Instructions

- Simply combine pistachios, chopped garlic, vegan Parmesan, olive oil, and basil in the bowl of a food processor. Season with salt and pepper and run your food processor until everything is combined and blended smoothly.

Nutrition Information

- Calories: 299| Total Fat: 29g| Saturated Fat: 4.6g| Trans Fat: 0g| Unsaturated Fat: 7g| Cholesterol: 0mg| Sodium: 0.8mg| Carbohydrates: 6.4g| Fiber: 1.3g| Sugar: 1g| Protein: 3.1g

41.Spaghetti Casserole

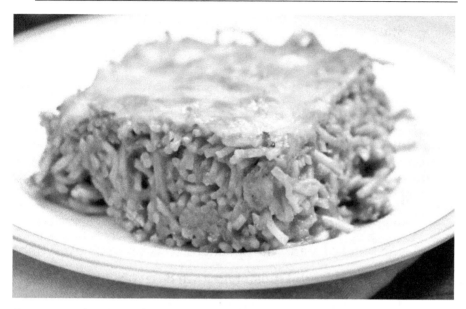

Serves: 4 | Prep Time: 10 Minutes | Cook Time: 20 Minutes |
Total Time: 30 Minutes

Ingredients

- 10 oz spaghetti (use gluten-free pasta, if you want)
- 16 oz marinara sauce
- 3 cloves garlic minced
- 1/2 cup vegan cream cheese
- 1/2 chopped onions
- 1 cup vegan cheese shreds
- Salt, pepper to taste

Instructions

- Start by cooking your spaghetti according to the package directions. After cooking, remove them from your pot.
- Heat a bit of oil or vegetable broth, add chopped onions, minced garlic, optional chopped bell pepper, and fry for around 2 minutes. Give the spaghetti sauce aka marinara, vegan cream cheese to the pot and season with salt and pepper. Cook for 3 minutes more until warm, add optional extras, if you like, cooked chickpeas, Italian seasoning.
- Next and last add the spaghetti back and mix everything until combined. Transfer all to an 8x11 inch casserole dish. Then sprinkle vegan cheese shreds over it and bake for around 10 minutes at 415Â°F.
- Serve on plates or bowls.

Nutrition Information

- Calories: 204| Total Fat: 11.8g| Saturated Fat: 6g| Trans Unsaturated Fat: 0.8g| Sodium: 237mg| Carbohydrates: 16.1g| Fiber: 3.6g| Sugar: 7.5g| Protein: 10g

42.　Instant Pot Spaghetti With Simple Tomato Sauce

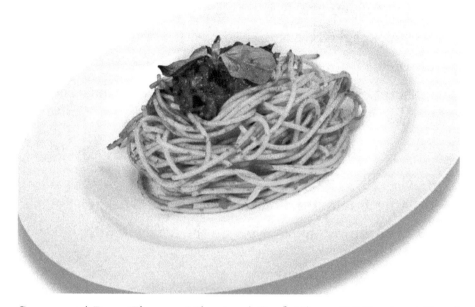

Serves: 4 | Prep Time: 5 Minutes | Cook Time: 8 Minutes | Total Time: 13 Minutes

Ingredients

- 10 oz spaghetti (i used gf)
- 2 tbs garlic powder
- 4 tsp italian herbs
- 24 oz marinara sauce
- 1 15 oz can light coconut milk
- 3/4 cup water
- 1/4 cup nutritional yeast, optional
- Salt, pepper to taste

Instructions

- Add all the ingredients, including the optional nutritional yeast if you like, to your instant pot. Make sure to break your spaghetti in half, season with salt and pepper.
- Dont stir the ingredients, just add everything. Also, make sure your pasta is complete covered with liquid, otherwise use a spoon to push your spaghetti down.
- Seal your instant pot, use the manual mode, and set it to high pressure and 8 minutes cooking time.
- After 8 minutes of cooking time, use quick release, and open the instant pot. Now stir the spaghetti with the sauce.

Nutrition Information

- Calories: 438| Total Fat: 11.9g| Saturated Fat: 8g| Trans Fat: 0g| Unsaturated Fat: 2.7g| Cholesterol: 0mg| Sodium: 69mg| Carbohydrates: 69.9g| Fiber: 5.7g| Sugar: 11.6g| Protein: 12.8g

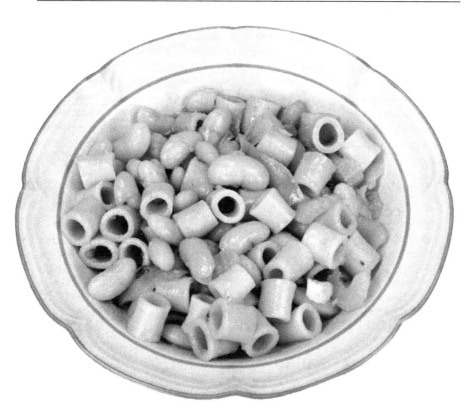

Serves: 6 | Prep Time: 5 Minutes | Cook Time: 15 Minutes | Total Time: 20 Minutes

Ingredients

- 2 cups pasta (I used gluten-free)
- 4 cloves garlic, minced
- 5 cups vegetable broth
- 28 oz marinara sauce
- 1 cup bell pepper

- 15 oz white beans
- Salt, pepper to taste

Instructions

- Start with a large pot. Heat a bit of oil or vegetable broth. Add bell pepper, garlic, and optional onions and fry everything for around 4 minutes.
- Now add uncooked pasta, vegetable broth, marinara, and cook all for around 12 minutes.
- Finally, add the white beans. Seasoning with salt and pepper, optional garlic powder, and Italian seasoning.
- Serve on plates or in bowls and sprinkle with optional vegan Parmesan.

Nutrition Information

Calories: 285| Total Fat: 3g| Saturated Fat: 0.6g| Unsaturated Fat: 1g| Sodium: 173mg| Carbohydrates: 52g| Fiber: 7g| Sugar: 11g| Protein: 11g

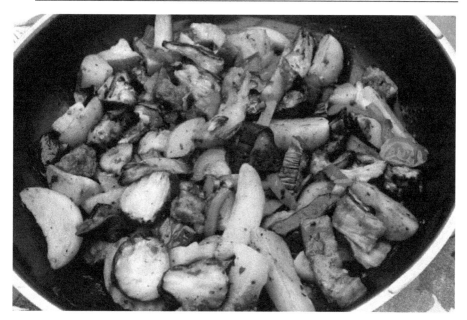

Serves: 4 | Prep Time: 5 Minutes | Cook Time: 30 Minutes | Total Time: 35 Minutes

Ingredients

- 1 lb gnocchi (I used gluten-free)
- 4 cloves garlic, minced
- 4 cups mixed vegetables (I used zucchinis, eggplants, tomatoes, bell pepper, onions)
- 1/3 cup olive oil, divided
- 2 Tbs balsamic vinegar
- Salt, pepper to taste

Instructions

- On a sheet pan mix the veggies like zucchinis, onions, eggplants, tomatoes, and bell pepper with 1/4 cup olive oil, minced garlic, and balsamic vinegar. Optionally you can also add maple syrup and herbes de Provence. Season with salt and pepper.
- Furthermore, on the same sheet pan, mix gnocchi with the rest of the olive oil and also season with salt and pepper.
- Finally, bake everything for around 20 minutes at 410°F. Serve on plates or in bowls.

Nutrition Information

- Calories: 465| Total Fat: 20g| Saturated Fat: 3g| Unsaturated Fat: 15g| Sodium: 63mg| Carbohydrates: 62g| Fiber: 7g| Sugar: 6g| Protein: 13g

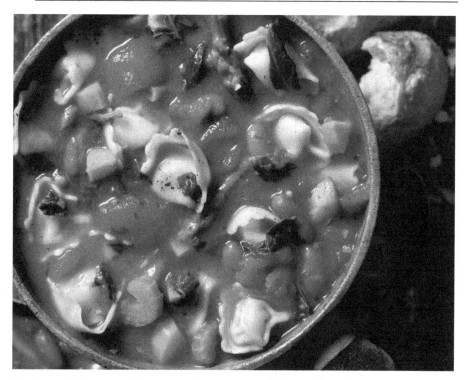

Serves: 6 | Prep Time: 5 Minutes | Cook Time: 15 Minutes | Total Time: 20 Minutes

Ingredients

- 1 lb vegan tortellini (I used Gf)
- 28 oz marinara sauce
- 3 cups vegetable broth
- 8 cloves garlic, minced
- 2 Tbs Italian seasoning
- 2 cups vegetables (I used onions, carrots, celery, leek, peas)

- Salt, pepper to taste

Instructions

- Heat a large pot with a bit of oil or vegetable broth. Add vegetables, garlic and fry everything for around 5 minutes.
- Next add vegetable broth, tomato sauce, Italian seasoning, and vegan tortellini. If you want also give the optional white beans to the mix. Season with salt and pepper and cook for around 8 minutes. If the tortellini aren't done yet, let simmer until they are.
- Serve in bowls and sprinkle optional with a good pinch of vegan Parmesan.

Nutrition Information

- Calories: 249| Total Fat: 6g| Saturated Fat: 2g| Trans Fat: 0g| Unsaturated Fat: 2g| Cholesterol: 0mg| Sodium: 100mg| Carbohydrates: 38g| Fiber: 4g| Sugar: 8g| Protein: 9g

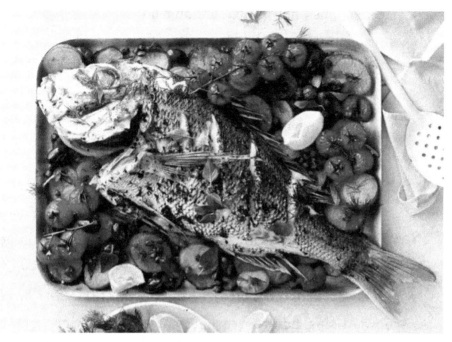

Prep Time: 25 Mins | Cook Time: 1 Hour | Serving: 8

Ingredients

- 400g cherry truss tomatoes
- 2/3 cup dry white wine
- 2 tablespoons lemon juice
- 4 garlic cloves, crushed
- 2 teaspoons ground coriander
- 1 teaspoon sweet paprika
- 2/3 cup extra virgin olive oil
- 1kg red-skinned potatoes, cut into 1cm slices
- 2/3 cup fresh oregano leaves, plus extra to serve

- 2/3 cup fresh dill sprigs, plus extra to serve
- 2 teaspoons finely grated lemon rind
- 1 teaspoon caraway seeds
- 1.5kg whole cleaned snapper
- 1/3 cup kalamata olives
- 2 tablespoons drained capers, rinsed
- Lemon wedges, to serve

Instructions

- Preheat oven to 200C/180C fan-forced. Grease a large baking tray with sides.
- Remove half of the tomatoes from the vine. Place in a large bowl. Using hands, crush tomatoes. Add wine, lemon juice, garlic, coriander, paprika, and 1 tablespoon oil. Season with salt and pepper. Stir to combine. Add potato. Toss to combine. Place potato mixture on prepared tray. Bake for 30 minutes.
- Meanwhile, place oregano, dill, rind, caraway seeds, and remaining oil in a small food processor. Season with salt and pepper. Process until finely chopped. Make 4 slits on each side of the fish. Rub dill mixture in the cavity and slits of fish. Place fish on potato mixture. Bake for 15 minutes.
- Cut remaining tomatoes into small portions. Add tomatoes, olives, and capers to the tray. Bake for a further

15 minutes or until fish is cooked through. Sprinkle with extra herbs. Serve with lemon wedges.

Nutritional Value

- Energy: 1503 Kj| Fat Total: 11.5g| Saturated Fat: 2.1g| Fibre: 4.8g| Protein: 42.3g| Cholesterol: 114mg| Sodium: 351mg| Carbs: 16.1g

Roasted Mediterranean Vegetables With Feta And Olives

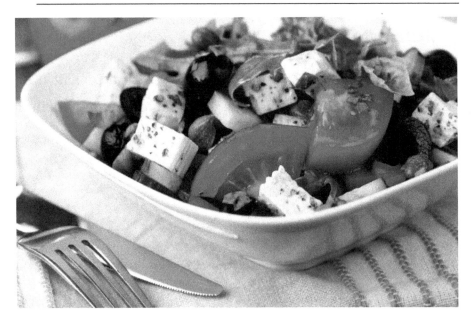

Prep Time: 10 mins | Cook Time: 25 mins | Servings: 4 serves

Ingredients

- 600g packet frozen Mediterranean vegetable mix
- 1 lemon, cut into wedges
- 1 red onion, cut into wedges
- 100g Greek feta, roughly crumbled
- 1/3 cup pitted kalamata olives
- 1 tablespoon red wine vinegar
- 2 tablespoons extra virgin olive oil
- 50g baby rocket

Instructions

- Preheat oven to 200C/180C fan-forced. Line a large roasting pan with baking paper. Place frozen vegetables and lemon in a prepared pan. Scatter with onion, feta, and olives. Bake for 20 to 25 minutes or until golden and tender.
- Meanwhile, whisk vinegar and oil together in a small bowl. Season with salt and pepper.
- Add rocket to vegetables. Toss to combine. Transfer to a platter. Serve with dressing.

Nutritional Value

- Energy: 1442 Kj| Fat Total: 22.2g| Saturated Fat: 7.2g| Fibre: 4.5g| Protein: 8.9g| Cholesterol: 17mg| Sodium: 889mg| Carbs : 24.4g

48.   Barbecue-Roasted Mediterranean Vegetables

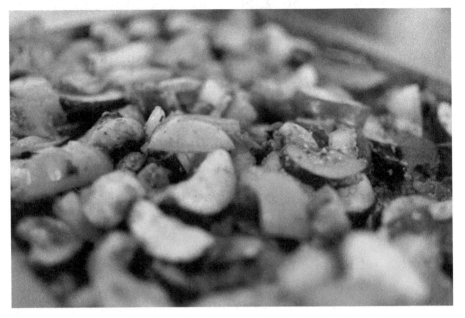

Prep Time: 20 Mins | Cook Time: 25 Mins | Serving: 4 Serves

Ingredients

- 1/2 x 350g tub marinated fetta
- 1 small red capsicum, halved, cut into 8 wedges
- 4 baby eggplant, halved lengthways
- 2 small zucchini, quartered lengthways
- 250g cherry tomatoes
- 4 garlic cloves, unpeeled
- 1/2 cup mixed marinated olives
- 4 x 5cm strips lemon rind
- 8 sprigs of fresh oregano, plus extra leaves to serve

- 2 tablespoons lemon juice
- Lemon wedges, to serve
- Select all ingredients

Instructions

- Preheat a barbecue hotplate on high heat.
- Drain fetta, reserving 1/3 cup marinating oil. Place capsicum, eggplant, zucchini, tomato, garlic, olives, lemon rind, and oregano sprigs in a bowl. Add lemon juice and reserved marinating oil. Season with salt and pepper. Toss to combine.
- Cut 4 x 50cm pieces of foil. Top each with a 20cm piece of baking paper. Spoon 1/4 of the vegetable mixture onto the center of each stack. Fold up edges of foil to enclose vegetables, scrunching foil at the top to seal. Place on a hotplate. Cook for 20 to 25 minutes or until tender and beginning to char.
- Place parcels on serving plates. Carefully open (steam will escape from parcels). Sprinkle with feta and extra oregano. Serve with lemon wedges.

Nutritional Value

- Energy: 1524 Kj| Fat Total: 33.1g| Saturated Fat: 8.9g| Fibre: 5g| Protein: 8g| Cholesterol: 12mg| Sodium: 691mg| Carbs: 6.6g

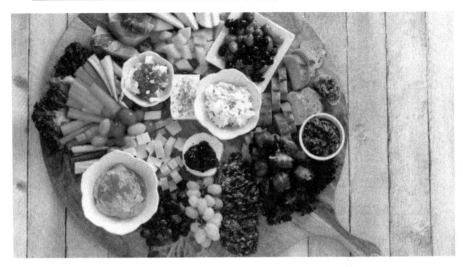

Prep Time: 15 Mins | Cook Time: 45 Mins | Servings: 6 Serves

Ingredients

- 2 tablespoons olive oil
- 1 garlic clove, crushed
- 1 long baguette, thinly sliced
- 200g marinated olives
- 200g thinly sliced mortadella
- 300g piece baked ricotta

Caponata

- 2 tablespoons olive oil
- 1 medium red onion, thinly sliced
- 1 yellow capsicum, thinly sliced
- 1 red capsicum, thinly sliced

- 1 baby eggplant, sliced
- 1 tablespoon red wine vinegar
- 400g can crushed tomatoes
- 2 teaspoons caster sugar

Instructions

- **Make Caponata:** Heat oil in a large, deep frying pan over medium heat. Cook onion and capsicum for 5 minutes or until softened. Add eggplant. Cook for 10 minutes or until softened. Add vinegar, tomatoes, and sugar. Bring to the boil. Reduce heat to low. Simmer for 20 minutes or until slightly thickened.
- Preheat oven to 220°C/200°C fan-forced. Line a baking tray with baking paper. Combine oil and garlic in a small bowl. Arrange bread slices, in a single layer, on a prepared tray. Brush with oil mixture. Bake for 10 minutes or until lightly browned.
- Arrange olives, mortadella, ricotta, and garlic croutons on a platter. Serve with Caponata.

Nutritional Value

- Energy: 2044 Kj| Total Fat: 29.6g| Saturated Fat: 8.6g| Fibre: 4.9g| Protein: 16.2g| Cholesterol: 45mg| Sodium: 979mg| Carbs: 38.7g

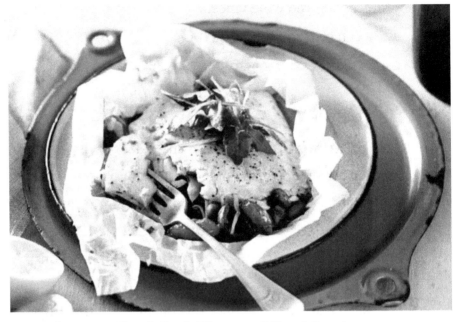

Prep Time: 15 Mins | Cook Time: 20 Mins | Servings: 4

Ingredients

- 400g can borlotti beans, rinsed, drained
- 200g grape tomatoes, halved
- 1 leek, cut into matchsticks
- 55g (1/3 cup) pitted kalamata olives, halved
- 1 1/2 tablespoons chopped fresh continental parsley
- 1 tablespoon drained baby capers
- 2 garlic cloves, thinly sliced
- 3 teaspoons extra virgin olive oil
- 4 (about 200g each) firm white fish fillets

- 2 tablespoons lemon juice
- Baby rocket leaves, to serve

Instructions

- Preheat oven to 200C. Cut four 50cm lengths of baking paper. Combine the beans, tomato, leek, olive, parsley, capers, garlic, and half the oil in a bowl. Season with pepper.
- Divide the bean mixture among the sheets of paper. Top with the fish. Combine the lemon juice and remaining oil in a bowl. Drizzle over the fish. Season. Fold the 2 long sides of each sheet of paper over the filling to enclose. Tuck the short sides under to seal. Place on a baking tray. Bake for 15-20 minutes or until the fish flakes when tested with a fork.
- Divide the parcels among bowls and top with baby rocket.

Nutritional Value

- Energy: 1181 Kj| Total Fat: 9g| Saturated Fat: 2g| Fibre: 6g| Protein: 36g| Cholesterol: 108mg| Sodium: 531.97mg| Carbs (Sugar): 4g| Carbs (Total): 11g

CONCLUSION

An overview of the historical antecedents and recent increased interest in the Mediterranean diet is presented and challenges related to how to improve the sustainability of the Mediterranean diet are identified. Despite its increasing popularity worldwide, adherence to the Mediterranean diet model is decreasing for multifactorial influences – lifestyle changes, food globalization, economic, and socio-cultural factors. These changes pose serious threats to the preservation and transmission of the Mediterranean diet heritage to present and future generations. Today's challenge is to reverse such trends. A greater focus on the Mediterranean diet's potential as a sustainable dietary pattern, instead of just on its well-documented health benefits, can contribute to its enhancement. More cross-disciplinary studies on environmental, economic and socio-cultural, and sustainability dimensions of the Mediterranean diet are foreseen as a critical need.

A Mediterranean diet for beginners might seem hard or unfamiliar. Though there is not one defined Mediterranean diet, this way of eating is generally rich in healthy plant foods and relatively lower in animal foods, with a focus on fish and seafood. Following a Mediterranean diet involves making long-term, sustainable dietary changes. Generally speaking, a person should aim for a diet that is rich in natural foods, including plenty of vegetables, whole grains, and healthful fats.

In summary, this diet is also a lifestyle, where physical activity, family, and health are prioritized. It can also be super beneficial for weight loss and other health concerns. Adopting a Mediterranean diet can prevent heart disease and reduce your blood sugar levels by restricting added sugars, refined grains, and processed food. Fortunately, Mediterranean meals are quite popular, strong in flavor, and diverse in choices. Anyone who finds that the diet does not feel satisfying should talk to a dietitian. They can recommend additional or alternative foods to help increase satiety. At the end of the day, the Mediterranean diet is incredibly healthy and satisfying. You won't be disappointed.

Mediterranean Cookbook

Top Mediterranean Recipes with Low Salt, Low Fat and Less Oil

Danielle Berry

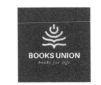

ISBN: 978-1-80252-598-4

CPSIA information can be obtained
at www.ICGtesting.com
Printed in the USA
LVHW081111210521
688044LV00013B/710